Praise for Functional Medic[...]
How to Be a Part of the Mo[...]
Transforming Heal[...]

There's no doubt that the evolution of medicine is going to rely highly upon health coaches to bring the right information and inspiration to life. Health coaches are what's needed to save American healthcare — and global health, for that matter. **If you are called to become a health coach and share your journey to inspire others, then you are called to change the world. This book is a powerful starting point, bringing the stories of others and how to use their success as a roadmap clearly into view.**

~ James Maskell, creator of Functional Forum, the world's largest integrative medicine conference

While it's easy to become frustrated with a system that does not help you truly heal your patients, it's obvious that becoming a health coach and employing Functional Medicine practices is a straight line to best practices and more success. **After decades of working with health coaches and practitioners at all levels and leading one of the largest communities in the space for those brand new to health coaching and seasoned veterans with vast credentials, I am confident this book will create huge inroads and help practitioners of all kinds to find new opportunities.**

~ J.J. Virgin, celebrity nutrition and fitness expert, four-time *New York Times* best-selling author

The paternalistic age of "I'm the doctor, you're the patient" is disintegrating. Every day people outside of the current healthcare model are gaining new power and insight through the astounding access to information that was not possible even 20 years ago. Health coaches are one of the few ambassadorships out there leading patients to take control over their own health by guiding them to cutting-edge information available for so many chronic conditions. **Self-empowerment in health has exploded, and health coaching is a powerful way to blaze new frontiers in helping people navigate health largely on their own, without conventional medical care, without hospitals and hospital procedures, without prescription drugs, and realized from the comfort of their kitchens and living rooms. Health coaches are a powerful part of where real healing is headed.**

~ Dr. William Davis, cardiologist, author of the *Wheat Belly* books

We all can feel a sense of pride for the US healthcare industry. Our technology has arguably created some of the most sophisticated diagnostic equipment in the world. Our doctors can diagnose the most difficult cases. But if we feel that sense of pride, then we must also recognize the complete failure in results. We must learn to differentiate technology success from clinical failure. The US healthcare system has been ranked #1 in technology but also ranked the worst in results of all industrialized nations for the fifth time.

A primary culprit for this embarrassment is the lack of compliance in lifestyle modification. Our doctors tell us to stop eating this, or do more of that, and we don't do it (for many reasons, but bottom line we just don't do it). Once you acknowledge these facts, the obvious component to getting better results is better compliance. Functional Medicine coaches are trained professionals that have dialed down how to work with the yabba, yabba, yabba of our minds — that voice that stops us from doing what we need to do. Diet, nutrition, exercise, attitude, mental roadblocks — when working with a FM coach, every obstacle is safe to address. And the more obstacles to lifestyle management that are addressed in a healthy, balanced way with your FM coach, the more likely you and your family are to develop the dynamic, vibrant health that is your birthright. Read this book. Learn where to find a FM coach, and thrive.

~ Dr. Tom O'Bryan, DC, CCN, DACBN, founder of theDr.com, internationally recognized speaker on gluten allergies and sensitivity

Functional Medicine Coaching:

How to Be Part of the Movement That's Transforming Healthcare

Sandra Scheinbaum, Ph.D.

Elyse Wagner, MS

Foreword by Dr. Mark Hyman

The education and information presented herein is intended for a general audience and does not purport to be, nor should it be construed as, specific advice tailored to any individual.

Do not disregard, avoid or delay obtaining medical or health related advice from your health-care professional because of something you may have read in this book. The use of any information provided in this book is solely at your own risk.

You should not rely on this information as a substitute for, nor does it replace, professional medical advice, diagnosis, or treatment. If you have any concerns or questions about your health, you should always consult with a physician or other health-care professional.

The health, wellness, fitness and information offered within this book are designed for educational purposes only.

Printed in the United States of America

First Printing, 2017

www.functionalmedicinecoaching.org

This book comes with one
FREE Functional Medicine health coaching session.
To set up your free session, text COACHING to
847-220-6353 or email
intakecoordinator@functionalmedicinecoaching.org
and instructions will be sent to you.

To the past, present and future students of the Functional Medicine Coaching Academy who are pursuing their passion and transforming healthcare.

Table of Contents

Disclaimer

The education and information presented herein is intended for a general audience and does not purport to be, nor should it be construed as, specific advice tailored to any individual.

Do not disregard, avoid or delay obtaining medical or health related advice from your health-care professional because of something you may have read in this book. The use of any information provided in this book is solely at your own risk.

You should not rely on this information as a substitute for, nor does it replace, professional medical advice, diagnosis, or treatment. If you have any concerns or questions about your health, you should always consult with a physician or other health-care professional.

The health, wellness, and fitness information offered within this book are designed for educational purposes only.

Foreword By Dr. Mark Hyman

In Functional Medicine Coaching, you'll be inspired by stories of positive transformation and healing. Allow me to tell you my story and why I'm so passionate about Functional Medicine, an approach to healthcare that's based on listening to the patient's story.

I'm the director of the Cleveland Clinic Center for Functional Medicine and the founder and medical director of The UltraWellness Center in Lenox, Massachusetts (www.ultrawellnesscenter.com).

Previously, I worked for almost 10 years as the co-medical director of Canyon Ranch in Massachusetts. I serve as chairman of the board of the Institute for Functional Medicine (IFM), the global leader in training providers in Functional Medicine, and authored more than a dozen books, including The *Blood Sugar Solution, The 10-Day Detox Diet*, and *Eat Fat, Get Thin*. I'm passionate about teaching for the Functional Medicine Coaching Academy and serving on its board of advisors, as I believe that health coaches trained in Functional Medicine represent the future of healthcare.

Trained in the conventional medical model, I not only mastered the demanding curriculum but thrived while in medical school. During that time, I ran four miles every day, practiced yoga, ate a whole-foods diet, and got enough sleep. But then I started working 36-hour shifts at the hospital. When I went to practice as a small-town family doctor in Idaho, I had a shortened schedule of only 80 hours per week. From Idaho, I went to work in China for a year, breathing in the coal-soaked, mercury-laden air. Then I went on to a crazy schedule of shifts in a Massachusetts inner-city emergency room.

So, it was not surprising that my body broke down. Severely fatigued, I couldn't pay attention, think clearly, or remember what my patients were saying to me. I couldn't sleep, my stomach was constantly bloated, my muscles ached and twitched, and I felt depressed and anxious. Doctor after doctor told me that there was nothing I could do. Some said I was depressed and recommended antidepressants; some suggested anti-anxiety drugs. My family doctor prescribed sleep medication. A neurologist told me I had ADD and needed stimulants. Others said I had chronic fatigue and fibromyalgia. I knew there was something really wrong; it wasn't just that I was depressed or stressed. Something was off.

Fortunately, I met Dr. Jeffrey Bland, the founder of The Institute for Functional Medicine. Through his teachings, I began to understand that the body is organized in a different way than I was taught in medical school. That training gave me the ability to diagnose thousands of different diseases. Functional Medicine views symptoms as the reflections of a few common interconnected imbalances. This approach addresses the whole system — the ecosystem of the body — not just how different parts operate independently from one another. Functional Medicine considers the whole person, not body parts.

Rather than a sudden onset, my condition was due to a long series of exposures to toxins, stress, and infection. The trail led back to mercury poisoning from living in China, eating endless tuna fish sandwiches as a child, and having a mouthful of "silver," or mercury fillings. I was also missing a key gene needed to detoxify mercury, which compounded the problem. Years of sleepless nights while working in the emergency room destroyed my body's rhythms, which I tried to bolster with espressos, chocolate chip cookies, and pints of Chunky Monkey ice cream. The straw that broke the camel's back was ingesting something that infected my gut while on a wilderness trip. Empowered by this new understanding of systems biology, I slowly put myself back together, working to correct the fundamental imbalances that are the cause of all disease.

As a result of my personal journey back to health through Functional Medicine, I became passionate about applying these principles in my work with patients. Rather than treating disease, I applied the science of creating health. I started to rethink the concept of illness, and by understanding the underlying biology through the science of Functional Medicine, my view of healthcare fundamentally changed.

The road map I was given in medical school to navigate through the territory of illness was the wrong map. I was taught to diagnose disease and then assign standardized treatments, no matter who was suffering. I was trained according to the dogma of separate medical specialties. For heart problems you see the cardiologist, for stomach problems you see the gastroenterologist, for joint pain you see the rheumatologist, for skin problems you see the dermatologist, and so forth. Using this map can send conventional doctors in the wrong direction.

A new road map has emerged for how the human body works and how to treat illnesses — mental or physical. Rather than based on the traditional ways of naming and diagnosing disease, this new road map is based on the underlying, core, interlocking physiological systems that underlie all disease.

Not only are symptoms such as joint pains, skin rash, constipation, and depression all connected, but the only way to alleviate these symptoms and reverse chronic disease is by using this new map, as it allows us to see how everything is connected. Functional Medicine offers this new road map that leads the way out. Functional Medicine applies the science of systems biology and represents a fundamental change in thinking about illness and the human body. Unlike conventional medicine, Functional Medicine personalizes treatment based on a patient's unique needs. We treat the soil and the terrains, not the plant.

I consider myself a medical detective who hunts down clues and explores the entire landscape of human biology. As a Functional Medicine doctor, I could relate thousands of patient success stories. I remember one patient who was sick since the age of nine and struggled for many years. Suffering from colitis, skin rashes, mood disorders, and fatigue, she was unable to work due to her autoimmune conditions. My treatment was simple: I addressed her gut issues with an elimination diet and gave her probiotics and simple nutritional support. When we addressed the underlying root causes of her conditions, she got better in a remarkably short period of time.

Another story involves a patient with schizophrenia who was being treated by a conventional physician with a psychiatric drug. I discovered that she suffered from Lyme disease, which was affecting her brain. She didn't need antipsychotic drugs; she needed antibiotics. I could also tell stories of patients with 40-year histories of migraines who were headache-free when they stopped eating certain foods or eliminated the mercury or other toxins that were contributing to their symptoms. It's been a powerful experience for me to see these and so many other transformations through Functional Medicine.

Rather than isolated anecdotes, stories of remarkable transformation and reversal of chronic disease repeat themselves over and over in medical practices based on Functional Medicine. These success stories happen because Functional Medicine identifies and addresses the underlying factors driving illness.

At the Cleveland Clinic Center for Functional Medicine, the first of its kind at an academic medical center, we've seen explosive growth. We quickly outgrew our space and opened an expanded facility in 2017. We started with two physicians and expanded to six, but still can't keep up with the demand. We can't hire fast enough. There are roughly 3,000 patients on the waiting list for appointments. In 2016, there were 4,200 visits. In 2017, we anticipate 14,000. The Center has seen patients from 17 countries and 42 states.

Our integrative team consists of doctors, nutritionists, nurses, and health coaches. During their first visit, patients spend an hour with a physician, an hour with a nutritionist, and 15 to 30 minutes with a health coach. The Center also has a space for group medical visits where patients can learn from one another. By fostering collaboration, we took away the hierarchy between physicians, nurses, nutritionists, and health coaches. Everyone on the team works collaboratively and listens to one another.

Why the rapidly expanding growth of Functional Medicine? People are understanding that there are underlying causes driving chronic illness that we need to deal with, and that there are limits to the potential for drugs and surgery to treat these conditions. Consumers want a different kind of care and are increasingly turning to Functional Medicine. On The Institute for Functional Medicine's website (www.functionalmedicine.org), you can search "Find a Practitioner" to locate a healthcare professional trained in Functional Medicine. In 2016, over one million people used this feature to find practitioners. At the present time, we pay for volume in health care instead of value. Functional Medicine will be a key part of the solution.

As the field of Functional Medicine continues to experience explosive growth, it will become increasingly more important to have health coaches trained in Functional Medicine principles. In this new paradigm shift for preventing and reversing chronic illness, health coaches play a crucial role. A Functional Medicine health coach can provide the tools and help patients find the motivation to apply this approach in their daily lives. Health coaches are uniquely suited to provide the crucial support and guidance that patients need to make diet and lifestyle changes.

Initiating and sustaining these changes can be challenging. If I say "take a pill," that's easy. But if I say "change your lifestyle or eat differently," those are difficult changes to make. People do better when they have support. I know this from firsthand experience.

I volunteered to do relief work in Haiti after the earthquake in 2010 and had the opportunity to meet Paul Farmer. He trained over 11,000 community health workers around the world, working in challenging locations such as Rwanda. Based on Dr. Farmer's experiences, I realized that people could accompany each other to health. Individuals were improving their health, not through better drugs or surgery, but by the power of peer-to-peer support. With this model, we can turn healthcare upside down. I want to train an army of Functional Medicine health coaches to go forth into communities, acting in a sense as upgraded health workers. At the Cleveland Clinic, I hope to expand services and build community-based programs for population health, providing access to Functional Medicine for thousands, even hundreds of thousands, of patients. Community healthcare represents the future, and we're going to need a lot of coaches to help us get there.

Health coaches teach people how to change their diets and live better, more fulfilling lives. They do not act as experts, but educated in Functional Medicine principles and nutrition, they have enough information to guide clients to make better choices and change habits. Coaches provide the key ingredient: social support. The coach, rather than acting as the expert, empowers the client to take charge of his/her health, and the two work as a team. Essentially, individuals engage with coaches to support them, either individually or in groups. With this type of teamwork, individuals can transform their behavior. They can receive feedback and be held accountable. Health coaches have to be integrated into every facet of the healthcare system, beginning in the community. The Functional Medicine movement cannot succeed without Functional Medicine health coaches, as inspiring behavior change is necessary if people are to actually get better. I can tell my patients what to do, but if they don't do it, my advice doesn't matter.

As a physician, scientist, and educator, I have struggled to find a comprehensive solution: a manifesto, a call to action, and a plan for us as individuals, families, communities, schools, workplaces, and faith-based groups to "take back our health." A diverse community-based movement is the only way to effectively reverse this epidemic of chronic disease. Conventional medicine is not equipped to deal with the tsunami of chronic diseases that we face. We need to decentralize and democratize healthcare, get it out of the doctors' offices and hospitals, and put it in different kinds of settings. These can include local community centers, churches, schools, corporations, fitness centers, and even the produce section of grocery stores, where health coaches can play a crucial role in transforming healthcare through education about "food as medicine."

My vision for the future is that Functional Medicine will be integrated into every aspect of healthcare. A true continuum of care would range from working with a community-based Functional Medicine health coach on diet and lifestyle changes, to seeing a Functional

Medicine practitioner, to acute care medicine such as surgery, when needed. Functional Medicine is about changing the way we do medicine and the medicine we do. The way we do medicine supports health coaching, as coaching represents the community base of prevention.

Health doesn't happen in the doctor's office; health happens where people live. We need to have health coaches take people shopping, go into their kitchens and cook a meal with them, and show them how to do the simple things that will ensure success. I can tell patients to "go eat hemp seeds," but if they don't know what hemp seeds are, that advice doesn't help. We have to bridge the gap, and I think health coaches are that bridge.

Health coaching is growing tremendously. Insurance companies and corporations are using health coaches, and hospitals are starting to use them. In Functional Medicine, there's no way we can do what we do without health coaches. They will be the future of how we create a successful, financially stable, and clinically effective healthcare system. I think it's an awesome moment in healthcare, and we're just at the beginning of a transformation in the health coach movement, particularly Functional Medicine health coaches. They're going to be critical for the future of healthcare.

I have an extraordinary job. I have the privilege of caring for people, being of service every day, and using my mind, experience, and knowledge to guide my patients toward greater well-being. As the chairman of the board of directors of the Institute for Functional Medicine, I am part of the transformation of medical education and practice that will change our notions about the treatment of disease. Most medicine of the future will not be about directly treating illness. Instead, it will be about creating health. Disease simply goes away as a side effect of creating health. I want to provide a clear solution for people to practice self-care. Health coaches will be a major part of the solution.

Functional Medicine provides a personalized road map for the journey back to health. Functional Medicine health coaches accompany patients on that journey. What if I had worked with a Functional Medicine health coach when I was ill many years ago? My coach would have educated me about how my lack of sleep, my gluten, dairy, and high-sugar diet, and my mercury toxicity were contributing to my symptoms. He/she would have helped me set realistic goals for behavior change, and we would have agreed on how I could be held accountable. Through this transformative experience, I would have become aware that I had the power to feel better.

What do you think derails someone from achieving their best health? Lack of preparation? Lack of willpower? Lack of resources? The number one obstacle people face on their journey toward better health is lack of support. Everyone wants to get healthy, but we all need someone to hold us accountable and to ask the right questions. We need someone to cheer us on and help us create a plan to achieve our goals. That is where a coach with the right training and the heart of a teacher comes in.

I include health coaches in all of my online programs and my programs at The UltraWellness Center and the Cleveland Clinic Center for Functional Medicine. Having health coaches on my team ensures that each and every individual gets healthy and, more importantly, stays healthy. Coaches bridge the gap between practitioners and patients, empowering people to take control of their wellness and reach their health goals.

I believe in health coaching so much that I started working with one of the best health coaching training programs available — the Functional Medicine Coaching Academy (FMCA). In collaboration with the Institute for Functional Medicine, my friends at FMCA created a completely online, year-long program that prepares students for a career as a Functional Medicine Certified Health Coach.

As a member of FMCA's board of advisors, I'm a strong proponent of the power of this program to transform the lives of students and the lives of the people they, in turn, coach. I believe in it so much that I had my own staff coaches complete the program.

Functional Medicine addresses the underlying causes of disease, using a systems-oriented approach and engaging both patient and practitioner in a therapeutic partnership. FMCA's comprehensive curriculum integrates the art of coaching with the principles of Functional Medicine, nutrition as medicine, the psychology of eating, mind-body medicine, and positive psychology.

If you've ever considered taking your career to the next level and participating in something that has an even greater potential to transform your life and the lives of others, I highly recommend the Functional Medicine Coaching Academy.

~ Dr. Mark Hyman

Introduction

"We need to move beyond asking what drug will treat the symptoms, and instead ask what mechanism creates altered function or systemic physiological change." — Dr. Jeffrey Bland, co-founder, the Institute for Functional Medicine; founder, Personalized Lifestyle Medicine Institute

How do we define health? In 1946, the World Health Organization stated that health is a state of complete physical, mental, and social well-being, not merely the absence of disease. The emerging field of Functional Medicine directly addresses the restoration of health by looking for common factors among various symptoms and diagnoses that can be improved (all the way down to the cellular level) through diet and lifestyle intervention. This model reaches beneath symptoms to restore function and generate momentum toward health. This moves us away from a model in which medicine's purpose is to treat chronic disease and into a model in which we heal the patterns that cause chronic disease.

Dr. Jeffrey Bland, widely recognized as the father of Functional Medicine, describes chronic diseases as those conditions or ailments that make you sick and never really go away. Their nature is to stay and come back again and again. We can manage their effects and find occasional relief, but we're unable to zap them away as we can infectious diseases.

In a model in which we spend too much and get too little (Americans rank 26 among 34 developed nations' health outcomes, while spending two and a half times more than most developed nations), we're clearly not paying attention to the right inputs for wellness.

Too often, the patient care process ends when a diagnosis is determined and medication is recommended. Drugs are typically only prescribed when the problem is acute or persistent enough to warrant intervention, leaving the early and often reversible stages of illness ignored. However, the Functional Medicine approach reverses this acute care model. The diagnosis becomes the beginning of the journey, and the patient's past and continuing stories represent the central drivers.

Today, almost half of all American adults suffer from at least one chronic illness. The Centers for Disease Control and Prevention estimates that managing these illnesses accounts for some 78 percent of the nation's health expenditures. A 2011 study by the World Economic Forum projected that by the year 2030, the cost of chronic illness treatment worldwide will exceed $47 trillion. That is why the time for Functional Medicine and Functional Medicine health coaches is now.

In this book, you'll discover how a Functional Medicine approach can restore health in a surprisingly short period of time. You'll discover how Functional Medicine health coaches blend the science-based principles of positive psychology and Functional Medicine with the art of coaching to help people create well-being. You'll read stories of coaches and their clients and learn how this dynamic process transforms the lives of both. Finally, you'll learn how you can wake up every morning thrilled to work in a field aligned with your mission and purpose.

A Functional Medicine practitioner working side-by-side with Functional Medicine health coaches epitomizes a model that will transform healthcare. The success stories presented in this book demonstrate the power of addressing the root causes of chronic disease through Functional Medicine combined with the support of the coaching relationship.

As founders of the Functional Medicine Coaching Academy, from our past experiences working with clients and our personal healing journeys, we know that the person who listens to our story and helps us make positive changes acts as the catalyst for growth and transformation.

By applying the Functional Medicine and positive psychology principles personally, we experienced their remarkable ability to heal both mind and body. We've since dedicated our lives to sharing the power of these approaches with our community and the world.

We hope that this book serves as a gateway to your next step on the healing path, whether that's becoming a Functional Medicine health coach or finding your own personal coach.

Sandra's Story

In my mid-20s, I frequently rushed to the emergency room believing I was having heart attacks. My doctor diagnosed me with severe panic disorders and prescribed medication, but I decided the pharmaceutical route was not for me.

Fortunately, in my psychology doctoral program, I enrolled in a workshop about mind-body medicine that included breathing for relaxation. I applied the techniques I learned to control my panic and anxiety and discovered more and more physical and mental relaxation strategies I could call upon. That was almost 40 years ago. I haven't had a panic attack since.

Over the years, I continued to study mind-body medicine, gathering a variety of methods for achieving inner peace. Some of these came from cognitive-behavior therapy, others from mindfulness training and positive psychology. After I discovered the important connection between food and anxiety and between exercise and anxiety, I radically changed my diet and began to work out regularly. I became a yoga instructor. With each new step, I found greater well-being.

I soon discovered the Institute for Functional Medicine (IFM) and decided to attend one of their conferences. It changed my life. Here was a transformational way of thinking about chronic illness by looking at root causes rather than just naming a condition and prescribing a particular treatment.

Had I seen a Functional Medicine practitioner after my first panic attack, he/she would have created a timeline that chronicled my story, noting that I had a family history of anxiety, was bottle-fed, took a lot of antibiotics, was traumatized by the early death of my father when I was nine, was under great pressure to earn a college scholarship, developed a sugar addiction, lacked exercise, and was likely deficient in vitamin D, protein, and omega-3. He/she would have seen my poor digestive health, underactive thyroid, high blood glucose levels, and panic attacks as a matrix of interconnected dysfunctions rather than isolated conditions. My mouthful of mercury dental fillings and possible exposure to other heavy metals and contaminants would have raised a red flag about toxic load.

When explaining my story back to me, a Functional Medicine practitioner would have discussed the likelihood that a diet high in sugar, gluten, dairy, and diet sodas was fueling inflammation and creating disturbances in important metabolic pathways, setting my brain "on fire." He/she would have initiated a plan for healing my digestive tract, reducing the underlying inflammation, and even helping my cells produce energy more efficiently. This type of practitioner might have explained the value of incorporating mind-body strategies to not just stop a panic attack, but to create physiological changes on a cellular level. We would have treated the root causes rather than just the symptoms of my anxiety.

If I had worked with a Functional Medicine health coach, we might have focused on "what's right," not "what's wrong." I could have identified my character strengths, including my love of learning, my creativity, and my zest. When I did poorly in student teaching, derailing my childhood dream of becoming a teacher, a coach would have helped me define where I wanted to be in the future and formulate goals.

How would my mother's life have been better if she had worked with a Functional Medicine health coach? After my father's sudden death, she saw a psychiatrist who prescribed tranquilizers. But becoming a widow with no marketable skills trying desperately to make ends meet is not a disorder. A coach trained in Functional Medicine might have helped her see the connections between stress and the development of hypertension, taught her relaxation techniques, and shown her how to prepare healthier meal choices. Most importantly, with a coach as her ally, she could have used her character strengths to find a renewed sense of meaning and purpose by establishing new relationships and embarking on a rewarding career path.

After that first workshop, I enrolled in every course The Institute for Functional Medicine offered. I am proud to be a member of the first graduating class (and the first clinical psychologist) of Functional Medicine Certified Practitioners. Not only did discovering Functional Medicine change my life, it also transformed the way I work with patients. Educated in a Functional Medicine way of thinking, I combined the basic principles with mind-body medicine, cognitive-behavioral therapy, and positive psychology. In my two books about panic disorders — Stop Panic Attacks in 10 Easy Steps and How to Give Clients the Skills to Stop Panic Attacks — I describe the effectiveness of this integrative approach.

Elyse's Story

When I was 13 years old, I was constantly sick, often racing to the bathroom in the middle of class. On top of that, I was overweight. Although I didn't feel well physically, what hurt worse was my classmates' taunting nickname: "Obese Elyse."

I knew certain foods just didn't agree with me, but I really loved to eat. I come from a Jewish background where food, family, and love were deeply intertwined. My earliest memories are of cooking and eating with my family, especially my grandmothers. To me, food meant love. But I was feeling so tired and sick at age 13 that I knew something about the way I was eating had to change.

My family found a nutritionist who truly took the time to listen to me. She empowered me with the knowledge to change my diet from processed foods to whole foods, added nutritional supplements, and urged me to eat organic foods whenever possible to avoid toxins. I lost about 50 pounds in two months. Not only that, my hair and nails started to grow. I thought to myself, "Holy guacamole! Food is medicine!"

The transformation wasn't easy. However, the nutritionist continued to work with me to change some deep-seated values and behaviors around food. Making these changes made me realize what I wanted to do with my life: empower others to transform, just as that nutritionist had helped me. As I earned my undergraduate degree in nutrition, I became frustrated by the paradigm I was learning. The "calories in, calories out" model just didn't fit with what I had experienced personally. For me, it had been so much more. Where was the part about changing behavior? What about understanding and working with mindset, attitudes, belief, and motivators?

I found a program that blended both at Bastyr University in Seattle, where I earned my master's in Nutritional Sciences and Clinical Health Psychology. The program was amazing, both educationally and personally. But in my second year of graduate school, my body sent me painful, ugly signals that were impossible to ignore. My digestive problems were back, but worse. I was exhausted, and my thoughts were foggy. My health began to affect my grades. Right before my worried parents were about to ship me off to the Mayo Clinic, I decided to see a Functional Medicine doctor.

After a genetic test, I was diagnosed with celiac disease. (Other doctors had previously ruled it out when a blood test had come back negative.) I felt relieved to have a diagnosis but overwhelmed at how I needed to change my life. I left the office with a few handouts about celiac disease and gluten, but for the rest, I was on my own. I remember thinking, "How am I going to do this by myself?"

Confused, overwhelmed, and frustrated, I spent a good year trying to figure out how to transition my diet, emotions, and mindset. Along with personal changes, I had to educate my friends and family on the protocols of living a gluten-free existence. My journey led to writing Smoothie Secrets Revealed, a book on how smoothies can help heal your gut. As I struggled to learn how to live with an autoimmune disease, I kept thinking, "I wish I had someone to guide me." "What if I had a Functional Medicine health coach?"

Our Vision

I joined Sandra's psychology practice in the Chicago area in 2013. We both shared a passion for partnering with clients on their wellness journeys. One of our most rewarding experiences involved co-leading weekly meetings, held in the staff kitchen of an oncologist's office, for patients with chronic disease. We were delighted that the power of community provided individuals with a renewed sense of meaning and purpose so they could sustain their newfound healthy habits. What we witnessed in this group was the effectiveness of Functional Medicine coaching. Although we didn't know it at the time, this pilot program contained all the elements of what would become the Functional Medicine Coaching Academy (FMCA) curriculum.

Visionaries by nature, we dreamed about ways to expand our influence to help more people. IFM was the global leader in training Functional Medicine practitioners. Didn't these doctors need health coaches to help their clients make the difficult lifestyle changes recommended? What if we created an online course that would prepare coaches to work in Functional Medicine clinics? We wondered if IFM would be interested in collaborating with us to create this program.

IFM liked our proposal, and with their support as our collaboration partner, we launched the Functional Medicine Coaching Academy (FMCA) in 2015. Our year-long program allows students to learn from world-renowned IFM faculty and leaders in positive psychology and hone coaching skills by working with clients during a six-month, supervised apprenticeship. The program catalyzes students' personal transformations into Functional Medicine health coaches who can help others find the power within to change.

FMCA integrates the principles of Functional Medicine and functional nutrition with the principles of positive psychology. These ways of thinking about the human condition are remarkably similar — both address what we need to thrive. Functional Medicine posits a matrix of interconnections where an imbalance in one area leads to an imbalance in other areas. Three crucial components sit at the heart of the matrix: mental, emotional, and spiritual. The FMCA curriculum also incorporates mind-body medicine, the psychology of eating, and fundamentals of cognitive-behavior theory, all disciplines that Sandra has been passionate about in her 40-year career as a health psychologist.

We train coaches to partner with Functional Medicine doctors to create strong teams for patient care. Our dream is to see a Functional Medicine Certified Health Coach in every doctor's office. With each class of FMCA graduates, we get closer.

We hope you will be as moved and inspired by the following stories as we are. Each one, in its own way, shows the power of Functional Medicine health coaching to transform not just the client and the coach, but the health of everyone on the planet.

To a healthier world,
Sandra Scheinbaum & Elyse Wagner

Part 1: How Functional Medicine Can Help You

The rapidly growing field of Functional Medicine originated in response to a conventional care model designed to treat acute symptoms. A revolutionary way of thinking, Functional Medicine focuses on healing entire systems within the human body. Pioneers in the field, including Dr. Jeffrey Bland, Dr. David Jones, and Dr. Mark Hyman, started by asking questions such as:

- What if the "problem" isn't the problem at all? What if it's a symptom of the actual problem?
- Why do symptoms that have been treated recur in a body? Is something else going on?
- If we treat one area of the endocrine/digestive/cardiovascular system, what impact does it have on the other parts of the system? On the entire body?

These questions gave rise to the science-based principles that comprise Functional Medicine.

In Part 1 of this book, you'll learn how Functional Medicine practitioners interpret the body's signals for help. You'll become aware of the missing piece in the health puzzle — the piece that bridges the gap between doctor and patient and translates the doctor's clinical knowledge into the patient's practical application: the Functional Medicine health coach.

Throughout Part 1, you'll find opportunities to deepen your journey with Functional Medicine if you're curious about how to bring these principles into your life. You'll also find stories that connect you with the power of the Functional Medicine health coach in the "Make the Connection" sections at the end of each chapter. These true stories from our students and their clients showcase the impact of Functional Medicine health coaching principles in action.

It's our intention that by the end of Part 1, you'll not only gain an understanding of Functional Medicine but will be as convinced as we are that Functional Medicine health coaches are the necessary partners for anyone who wants to find greater wellness.

Chapter 1: What is Functional Medicine?

(And why everyone needs a Functional Medicine health coach)

"Functional Medicine is the wave of the future." — Dr. Mark Hyman, director, the Cleveland Clinic Center for Functional Medicine; director, The UltraWellness Center; chairman, the Institute for Functional Medicine

There is perhaps no stronger evidence for the power of Functional Medicine than the story of Dr. Terry Wahls, author of The Wahls Protocol and The Wahls Protocol Cooking for Life. Dr. Wahls ran marathons, climbed mountains, and had a busy practice as a physician and clinical professor of medicine at the University of Iowa Carver College of Medicine. Then she was diagnosed with multiple sclerosis, and at the age of 52, she was confined to a tilt wheelchair. She came to the realization that the conventional medicine she practiced in her own distinguished career had no treatments to halt her progressive decline.

Fortunately, she didn't accept her fate and drew upon her love of learning and perseverance to find the healing path. She began her journey toward wellness by adopting a Paleo diet, which involves removing all grains, legumes, dairy, refined sugar, and other processed foods. But the real answer came when she stumbled upon Functional Medicine. Here was an evidence-based approach that held promise for reversing autoimmune conditions such as multiple sclerosis.

Dr. Wahls enrolled in a Functional Medicine program and wrote that "although it was difficult at first, that Functional Medicine course taught me that I could improve the condition of my mitochondria and my brain cells. It gave me an entirely new way of thinking about brain health and how it relates to whole-body health. Although it wasn't the way I was trained, it made sense to me. It was all logical and scientifically-supported. It resonated with me as a doctor, but it also fit into the context of my experience as an MS patient."

By further refining her diet and lifestyle and adding supplements targeted to her unique needs, Dr. Wahls reversed her MS and now bikes to work each day. Her mission is to help others suffering from this debilitating condition by conducting research on the effectiveness of the Functional Medicine protocol that she created.

What Is Functional Medicine?

Functional Medicine looks at the pattern of dysfunction underlying chronic diseases and offers a model of care that can prevent or reverse such illnesses. It is based on the way our genes are stimulated and respond to our environment (what's going on around us and the kinds of behaviors we practice.) The guiding principle is that if we can change our environment and our behavior, we can change the way our genes perform.

A central piece of the "environment" is the patient's chosen lifestyle. An increasing amount of research demonstrates the therapeutic effectiveness of lifestyle interventions for the treatment of many chronic diseases. One major environmental factor that modifies gene expression is the individual's nutritional status. Nutrients can influence the expression of genes, the translation of the genetic message into active protein, and that protein's ultimate influence in controlling metabolic function.

This means that our genes do not predetermine our health. No single gene controls the presence or absence of chronic disease. Our pattern of health and illness is determined by how families of genes are expressed, and that expression can be influenced and altered by a range of lifestyle, diet, and environmental factors.

Evidence is now emerging of the complex interactions between genes and the environment in the causation of many diseases. We can change the way our genes get stimulated and the way they respond, and since genes regulate and direct biological functions, we can create health.

Functional Medicine practitioners adopt a flexible perspective on treatment approaches. The use of drugs or surgery does not disappear, but lifestyle interventions assume a primary role where appropriate. These are prioritized for their lower cost and because of their long-term role in the restoration of health and the prevention of disease.

"Personalized, preventative, and participatory" are the hallmarks that define Functional Medicine. Adherents believe that most chronic diseases are preventable and even reversible if a comprehensive individualized approach addressing genetics, diet, nutrition, environmental exposure, stress, exercise, and psychospiritual needs is implemented through collaborative care teams.

The Core Physiological Systems

Functional Medicine identifies seven core physiological processes that interconnect and define how we function. In the Functional Medicine paradigm, a breakdown of these seven will lead to a host of symptoms we currently link to chronic illness:

- Digestion and assimilation
- Detoxification
- Defense and repair
- Cellular communication
- Cellular transport
- Energy
- Structure

Chronic illness is a result of an imbalance in one or more of these core physiological processes. Such an imbalance is rooted in the interaction between lifestyle, diet, and environment and alters genetic function. Over time, that altered function is evidenced in specific symptoms that we collectively label a disease.

In the appendix, you'll find the Functional Medicine Matrix — aptly named, as each component of this interconnected web "talks to" every other area. Functional Medicine practitioners use the Matrix as a tool to help identify imbalances among the seven core processes. They recognize the importance of two areas of the Matrix: the five categories of modifiable lifestyle factors (described below) and the "heart," or center, of the Matrix — the mental, emotional, and spiritual components. These factors impact the core physiological processes, resulting in either altered function and the development of chronic illness or health maintenance and a state of balance.

Change Your Environment

By addressing the following modifiable lifestyle factors, we can bring our core physiological processes back into balance:

- Sleep and relaxation
- Nutrition and hydration
- Exercise and movement
- Social relationships
- Stress

These five factors are the "environment" that surrounds your genes. By changing the environment, you tell your genes to express themselves in a way that creates optimal health.

What Is Health Coaching?

Michael Arloski, PhD, an early proponent of wellness coaching, defines health coaching (interchangeably referred to as "wellness coaching") as the application of the principles of life coaching to the goals of lifestyle improvement for higher levels of wellness. This powerful model works because it is client-centered and focuses on finding meaning and purpose.

Health coaching must not be equated with health education. The two are quite different. We have wonderful programs geared to health promotion, but while people may desire to pursue healthier habits and know what to eat or how to exercise, they "just don't do it." Working with a coach can close the gap between intention and behavior.

Coaching provides a positive relationship that empowers the client to make lasting changes for better health and well-being. Most people experience a gap between knowing what they have to do and actually doing it. That's where coaching becomes relevant. Through inquiry, reflection on strengths, values, visions, and powerful dialogue, coaches supply invaluable fuel for their clients' transformation.

Health coaches work in a variety of settings, including hospitals, clinical practices, corporate wellness programs, insurance companies, spas, and private practices. Demand for their services is increasing. Yoga instructors, personal trainers, and allied healthcare professionals are becoming health coaches. Many practitioners are enrolling in coaching programs so they can add coaching to their existing skill sets. At the Functional Medicine Coaching Academy, we train physicians, nurses, dentists, psychologists, social workers, dieticians, chiropractors, acupuncturists, and massage therapists, to name just a few professions.

Although health coaching is a new field, it's growing rapidly, and both the healthcare industry and individual consumers are appreciating the value of this powerful model. Studies show that health coaches can help people manage chronic conditions (such as diabetes), lose weight and keep it off, increase movement and activity, and generally improve their physical and mental health. Employers appreciate how coaches can help bring down patient coverage costs and reduce claims. More and more medical centers and major hospitals are hiring health coaches, and many insurance companies offer coaching programs.

As the popularity of health coaching continues to grow, the need for certification and proper training increases, as well. It is vital that health coaches learn how to build trusting relationships, identify client values and desires, and know how to help each client transform his or her unique goals into actions that create lasting change and true health, wellness, and vitality.

The International Consortium for Health and Wellness Coaching (ICHWC), a voluntary team of leaders, together with the National Board of Medical Examiners, launched a National Board Certification for Health and Wellness Coaches. In September 2017, the ICHWC will offer its first certification exam. ICHWC has strict criteria and only allows graduates of approved health and wellness training programs to take the test. The Functional Medicine Coaching Academy is an approved school.

The objective of the certification is to provide minimum competency standards and assess mastery of the knowledge and skills essential to the practice of health coaching. National and international certification helps standardize and legitimize this missing piece of our healthcare system.
Through video conferencing platforms, a Functional Medicine health coach meets with clients in person, over the phone, or online, either individually or in groups. During the initial consultation, clients tell the

coach their story and talk about their vision for their future lives. For example, they might describe what their daily routine would look like if they had no pain or if they achieved their goal weight.

Then the client and the coach collaborate to set goals and determine how many coaching sessions may be appropriate to meet those objectives. Because coaching is a client-centered process, a coach does not set the goals but helps the client establish them through an inquiry process. A coach helps the client decide where he or she want to begin a unique journey toward better health. While the nonjudgmental coach may help a client brainstorm ideas, the client always arrives at his or her own conclusions. This is key to cultivating the client's sense of empowerment. In this way, the coach helps the client take charge of his or her life.

Next, the Functional Medicine health coach and the client work together to break the client's main goals into smaller, more achievable ones. Specific goals might be formulated around nutrition, hydration, exercise, relaxation, sleep, or social connections. Although the coach may know what areas need to be addressed, the client chooses what to work on and where to begin.

A Functional Medicine health coach educates and supports clients as they make important diet and lifestyle changes. But the process isn't just teaching clients to eat this and not that or to get more sleep and reduce stress. A vital component of the coaching process involves helping clients discover their own power to change. To do this, coaches use techniques rooted in positive psychology.

Positive psychology looks at how to nurture what is best within people to help them thrive. Coaches trained in this approach help clients discover their signature character strengths and use them to change behaviors, find well-being, and lead more meaningful lives.

It's important to note that a Functional Medicine health coach cannot take the place of a medical doctor, psychologist, or nutritionist. The coach does not make recommendations or write prescriptions; he or she educates, listens, and asks questions.

The Key to Functional Medicine Health Coaching

Making changes in modifiable lifestyle factors can be challenging. Education is not enough. Scare tactics fail. Coaches support clients as they make the difficult behavior changes required to prevent or reverse chronic disease. That's why an increasing number of Functional Medicine practitioners are adding coaches to their team.

To be effective, health coaching cannot just be about helping clients adhere to dietary plans or supplement regimens. We believe that the most important job of a Functional Medicine health coach involves creating a partnership with clients to discover the mental, emotional, and spiritual components that drive their motivation to heal. Coaches explore the heart of the Functional Medicine Matrix with clients.

Both from personal and clinical experience, we've seen that people change when their minds and hearts change — when their beliefs about what's possible for them change. For this reason, the Functional Medicine Coaching Academy's curriculum takes a deep dive into the principles of positive psychology. By helping clients leverage their strengths and connect to their will to heal and live, coaches become the ferrymen at the River Styx, helping clients reverse the journey from chronic degeneration toward the ability to thrive again.

Additionally, Functional Medicine health coaches act as a navigator through the web of practitioner care for chronic illness. To manage their symptoms, many patients with chronic illnesses face a gauntlet of a minimum of three to four doctors. Coaches often make the difference between "getting doctor's orders" and "following doctor's orders" by helping patients leverage their mental, emotional, and spiritual drivers.

In the coming chapters, you'll learn how Functional Medicine health coaches listen to, organize, and reframe clients' stories. By sharing their stories, clients understand the environments that triggered the onset of chronic disease and find the strengths to create wellness.

Prioritize the Client's Story

The importance of understanding the client's experience of his or her illness cannot be overemphasized. In a Functional Medicine approach, we prioritize listening to our clients' stories to gain insight into the environments that caused their genes to express themselves through patterns of chronic illness. Doctors often fail to pay attention to patients' concerns and miss important clinical information. Extensive research done within the context of conventional medical care reveals what most patients know: Doctors do not pay enough attention to what their patients say.

The first step in patient-centered care consists of eliciting patients' stories in a comprehensive manner. The role of Functional Medicine practitioners is to go beyond the diagnoses — to uncover the physical and social environments in which chronic diseases occur, including diet and lifestyle patterns. By actively listening to their patients' stories, they discover the antecedents, triggers, and mediators that underlie discreet symptoms and specific illnesses.

Integrate the Client's Story

After listening to the concerns that led each client to seek a consultation, the Functional Medicine practitioner asks questions that will identify the antecedents, triggers, and mediators that led to present and past health problems.

Antecedents

Antecedents consist of family history and events that occurred before, during, and immediately after birth. For example, a client is asked if his or her mother smoked during pregnancy, if he or she was born by Cesarean section, and if he or she was breast-fed. Practitioner and client talk about significant events that took place during the client's childhood, such as recurrent ear infections, bullying, or parental divorce.

Functional Medicine practitioners and coaches trust that clients can identify precipitating events that preceded the development of chronic illness.

According to Dr. Leo Galland, one of the early leaders in Functional Medicine, "They represent a boundary in time: before this event, the person was considered healthy; since the event, the person has become a patient." To uncover precipitating events, we ask, "When is the last time you really felt well for more than a couple of days at a time?" "During the six months preceding that date, did you experience major stress or make any significant changes in your life?"

Triggers

Triggers can be anything that results in the emergence of symptoms. Common triggers include microbes, drugs, allergens, foods, environmental toxins, and stressful life events. For most chronic illnesses, multiple interacting triggers can be identified.

Mediators

Mediators are ongoing factors that might be driving the current symptoms, such as lack of physical activity, poor dietary patterns, lack of sleep, environmental exposures, high stress load, and lack of meaning, purpose, or pleasurable experiences. There are typically many interacting mediators that perpetuate chronic illness, including a patient's beliefs about the disease. As you'll see, finding resiliency through character strengths can act as a positive mediator that interrupts disease progression.

While listening to a patient's story, Functional Medicine practitioners may ask questions to elicit the patient's beliefs about his or her illness, such as:

- What do you think has caused your problem?
- What do you most fear about your problem?
- How much control do you think you have over your symptoms?
- Are there people in whom you can confide?
- How satisfied are you with your marriage, your family, your friends, and your social life?
- How much support do you receive in dealing with your health problems?
- How often do you feel loved or cared for?

Organize the Client's Story: The Functional Medicine Approach

Functional Medicine involves a conscious synthesizing process that answers these questions: Who is this person? Why is he or she in pain? How can he or she thrive again? When piecing together the puzzle that each new client presents, the process of mapping symptomatology to the experiential timeline of a patient's life provides clues for the direction of healing.

But the Functional Medicine approach consists of more than hearing the client's story and the sequence of events in his or her life. It's about understanding the client's interpretation of these events. The Functional Medicine physician and Functional Medicine health coach work together to provide a road map for the client's healing journey. This map is further customized when the health coach adds the client's strengths to make the route accessible.

As you can see, in the Functional Medicine approach, there's a distinct focus on the client's entire life, not just his or her symptoms. In the life of the client, the Functional Medicine health coach functions as a bridge between the doctor's orders and the environment the client will modify to create healthy gene expression. In other words, the coach is the bridge between the client and his or her goal of optimal health.

We invite you into the world of Functional Medicine health coaching. In the remaining chapters of this book, we will guide you through a Functional Medicine approach to healing and provide stepping stones to wellness through tools that put the power to thrive in your hands. We will give you a taste of what it might be like to become (or work with) a Functional Medicine health coach.

Chapter 2: Tell Your Story

"Our minds influence the key activity of the brain, which then influences everything: perception, cognition, thoughts and feelings, personal relationships; they're all a projection of you." — Deepak Chopra, author, public speaker, alternative medicine advocate

The practice of Functional Medicine begins by listening to the patient's story. In this patient-centered care approach, individualized treatment plans are based on an understanding of the physiological, environmental, and psychosocial context within which each person's illness occurs.

While practitioners create a timeline of significant life events, including medical history and important milestones, Functional Medicine health coaches take the time to ensure that clients fully understand how modifiable lifestyle factors created and perpetuate current health challenges. Practitioner and coaches work together to identify ways to change stories by changing environments. Most importantly, coaches listen for opportunities to reframe the stories in light of the clients' unique strengths.

The Functional Medicine health coach facilitates the process of discovering the redemptive aspect to one's personal narrative. According to Dan McAdams, a psychologist at Northwestern University, there are two types of narratives we use to identify who we are: the redemptive story and the contamination story.

In the redemptive story, individuals describe the positive features of circumstances, consider the perspective of positive outcomes that may have come from challenging events, and share how they used strengths such as courage and perseverance to overcome obstacles.

McAdams describes the opposite of a redemptive story as a contamination story. In this version, people interpret their lives as going from good to bad. Those who tell contamination stories tend to be more depressed and anxious. They believe their lives are less meaningful than the lives of those who tell redemptive stories. Themes of stagnation, regression, helplessness, loneliness, and isolation mark the contamination story.

Nutritionist, fitness expert, and New York Times best-selling author JJ Virgin offers a striking example of creating a redemptive story, which she describes in Miracle Mindset: Show Up. Step Up. You Are Stronger Than You Think. This could have been a contamination story about how her life changed for the worse when her son almost died following a hit-and-run accident. Instead, she relates a redemptive story of courage, hope, and gratitude. Following a tragic event, Virgin transformed her life to one with renewed meaning and purpose, helping others find their own Miracle Mindset.

When a coach collaborates and listens to the client's story, together they can create the redemptive story. Even making very small edits to the story can have a profound impact on how clients view themselves and thus what they say and do to implement positive changes to improve their health.

The coach takes a strength history and asks clients to focus on times they used these strengths. The coach helps clients experience hope and appreciate that they are resilient, that they have unique contributions and potential, and that through exploring these values, they can strive for healthier, more meaningful lives and relationships. In this process, the coach acts as a collaborator.

In the appendix to this book, you'll find the Functional Medicine Timeline that Functional Medicine practitioners and health coaches complete when listening to a client's story. We invite you to create your own timeline. By engaging in this exercise, you'll get a holistic view of the onset of symptoms and identify the antecedents, triggers, and mediators that contributed to the development of any chronic condition. After filling in your timeline, review your story. Can you find elements that would make it a redemptive narrative? Add your strengths history, which you'll learn more about in Chapter 3.

Included in this book are stories relayed to us by Functional Medicine health coaches and clients that demonstrate the power of creating a redemptive narrative. The storytellers could have stuck with a version that involved accepting declining health and a poor prognosis, as they were frequently told by medical practitioners to accept such an outcome. But these brave individuals chose to write a different interpretation. They did so to help others find better health and well-being. Although the stories that follow may begin by describing pain, suffering, and loss, they are the opposite of contamination narratives. Instead, filled with resiliency, character strengths, empowerment, meaning, and purpose, they exemplify the power of a redemptive story.

We hope you will be inspired by these stories. All are true. All showcase the power of Functional Medicine and Functional Medicine health coaching.

Make the Connection: Functional Medicine and the Power in Your Story

Charmaine Cota, Indiana, USA

Three years ago, I was a newly certified personal trainer. And being new — to the industry and to my role — I was having trouble building a client base.

That's when I bumped into an old friend. She was a nutritionist and had just started working for Dr. Ellen Antoine, a Functional Medicine doctor. My first thought was that we could help each other build our client bases, so I asked my friend for an introduction. I had no idea what Functional Medicine was. And I had no idea Dr. Antoine would save my life.

Upon meeting, Dr. Antoine and I immediately loved each other's passion for the health and wellness of others. I started training her staff, and then one of her clients hired me as their corporate wellness director and executive personal trainer. Life was good.

Then my hectic work schedule and family life started to collide. A stroke left my mother mute and paralyzed, which caused "sibling stress" to go through the roof. My financial stress increased as well, with two kids entering Catholic high school and two kids in Catholic grade school. I was also in marital distress on crazy levels . . . that's what kicked my bucket over.

Things came to a head for me when we returned from a family spring break. After the long but easy 13-hour drive home, I couldn't get out of bed for three days. I felt like I had the flu, but I had no fever. I experienced slurred speech, poor memory, brain fog, migraines, and silent migraines. For months, I couldn't make it through the day without a nap. I'd have weeks of cramps like I was menstruating. I'd get bloated and have gas every time I ate. Visits to doctors provided no answers, and blood tests revealed nothing abnormal. I decided I needed to visit Dr. Antoine. She got me in right away, thank my lucky stars.

During my visit, we discussed my history, from birth to the present, including stress, family, marriage, finances, and job dissatisfaction. She also conducted comprehensive blood tests, which revealed a severe allergy to mold. A full home mold test divulged mold in my house; I had been exposed for the 14 years I had lived there. My toxin count was sky high, and Dr. Antoine also told me I had food sensitivities that were contributing to impaired digestion.

This new knowledge was hard to process. On the one hand, I was relieved to finally have some answers to what was going on in my body. But on the other hand, I could barely think straight, let alone absorb what the nutritionist was telling me I had to do next. At age 44, I was suddenly in the worst shape of my life.

Determined to recover from this health crisis, I started on Dr. Antoine's regimen: the supplements, the mold elimination diet, the gratitude journal, dry skin brushing, positive thinking, positive social situations, working on my marriage, and trying to get out of my moldy home. I did everything Dr. Antoine or her staff told me to do. I felt like they were the only ones who understood me and supported me.

Almost one year later, I have more energy and focus, the cramping and silent migraines are gone, and my toxin numbers have significantly reduced. I am focusing on my health and my family's health. We're making good choices — not just food, exercise, and environment choices, but choices that improve our mindfulness, as well.

Nancy Uston-John, Pennsylvania, USA
I honestly believe that all of the events in my life happened for a reason, and I am hoping my experiences will allow me to help others on their journeys. My story is one of autoimmunity.

Although I had been an active athlete since high school, I found myself in a state of fatigue after the birth of my second child in 2011. I chalked it up to being a tired mom of two who just needed more sleep. But a year later, after a round of antibiotics for a sinus infection, I found my digestion in the worst state ever. I was battling a host of symptoms, including brain fog, muscle soreness, joint pain, constipation, memory issues, hormonal issues . . . the list goes on.

I decided that enough was enough and visited a traditional doctor. After a few rounds of blood work, she said there was nothing wrong with me. She told me I was depressed and that I needed to get a hobby. I told her that I was not depressed but that I was going to be if I could not get back to living the way I knew I could.

My journey continued, and I visited four other doctors: naturopathic doctors, chiropractors, and a hormone specialist. The hormone specialist finally diagnosed me with Hashimoto's thyroiditis. Although my thyroid levels were in the normal range, my antibodies were literally off the charts.

My online research led me to Functional Medicine. I began working with a Functional Medicine doctor to repair my body. I learned I had various vitamin deficiencies, mitochondrial issues, food sensitivities, bacterial overgrowth . . . again, the list goes on. So I changed my diet, eliminated my intense workouts, considered true stress reduction for the first time in my life, and learned how past emotional traumas were affecting me. Since that time, my symptoms have been cut in half. Given several enormous personal losses I experienced during this past year, my turnaround is all the more impressive.

I truly believe in Functional Medicine's ability to get to the root of the problem. I want to help other people, especially those with chronic conditions, find the answers they seek, just as I have found mine. When I learned about the FMCA program, I knew that this is what I was meant to do.

Eileen Immerman, Wisconsin, USA

After reading Ultra-Metabolism by Dr. Mark Hyman, I realized my thyroid wasn't working right. This was maybe a year after I finished chemo. My internist had put me on a thyroid medication, and after losing a little weight initially, I stalled and couldn't lose any more. Up late one night (I was also dealing with insomnia), I googled Dr. Hyman's name, thinking, "I wonder if he teaches anywhere?" I found that he was leading an

Ultra Metabolism class in Massachusetts, near where he practices. Off I went.

At the class, I shared with Dr. Hyman that I had autoimmune rosacea and idiopathic thrombocytopenic purpura, a platelet autoimmune disorder that causes bruising all over the body. I was treating these conditions, but nothing was working. Dr. Hyman said, "You have a toxin in you and we have to figure out what it is." I said, "Well, how do I do that?" He replied, "You come see me." I called his office and got in the next day during his lunch hour. During the appointment, he drew labs, and within two or three weeks, we knew I had mercury toxicity.

I also had insulin resistance and high blood sugar. "Of course, you're hungry all the time," Dr. Hyman told me. "Anybody would be, with a fasting insulin this high. And until we get this mercury out of you, it's not going to straighten itself out." Within three weeks of beginning chelation treatment to remove the mercury, my platelets were climbing. My oncologist and hematologist were shocked. For the next five years, I stayed on chelation and got better and better.

I am convinced that the mercury set me up for my breast cancer. It changed my immune system to a point where my body was attacking my platelets and my thyroid. Dr. Hyman recognized the problem when no one else did. I wish that I could send every single physician in my town to a Functional Medicine training course.

———

As you can see, sharing one's story reveals personal strengths and a capacity to thrive, elements that play a critical role in the ability to heal. One common theme we celebrate in the redemptive story is the "enough moment."

This is the moment when the client decides that he or she is through suffering and is willing to do whatever it takes to feel better again.

We celebrate this moment because within it, varying combinations of hope, courage, self-awareness, and faith coalesce to help the client begin the process of telling a different story — the personal "strengths story."

Chapter 3: You Are Not Your Disease: Rewrite Your Story

"With everything that has happened to you, you can either feel sorry for yourself or treat what has happened as a gift. Everything is either an opportunity to grow or an obstacle to keep you from growing. You get to choose." — Dr. Wayne W. Dyer, New York Times best-selling author, self-development speaker

Functional Medicine health coaches help clients become the best version of themselves. In Positive Identities: Narrative Practices and Positive Psychology, Dr. Margarita Tarragona writes, "We can choose to embody, bring forth, or perform different ways of being, different versions of who we are."

This sense of possibility can initiate a process of growth and transformation. Coaches help clients choose which version is closest to their dreams, values, commitments, and the kinds of relationships they want to have, essentially helping them find new meaning in their life stories. Clients can choose their preferred way of "being" by using their character strengths.

The field of study that merges positive psychology and narrative practice with Functional Medicine principles is uniquely suited to preparing coaches to listen to and help reframe stories, an important element in the Functional Medicine approach to health coaching.

Positive Psychology

In 1999, Dr. Martin Seligman, then the president of the American Psychological Association, wanted to advance the science of character. He conceived the notion of positive psychology, a discipline focused on the positive aspects of the human experience. Until then, psychology focused on diagnosing and treating mental disorders. Dr. Seligman wanted to understand what contributed to a good life. He envisioned a new discipline with three essential components: positive emotions, positive traits, and positive organizations.

Dr. Seligman researched the factors that contribute to flourishing. The result was PERMA, the essential five elements that we need to thrive: **P**ositive emotions, **E**ngagement or flow, **R**elationships that are meaningful, a sense of **M**eaning and greater purpose, and **A**chievement or accomplishment. We find these pillars of well-being through character strengths.

Rather than attempting to negate a focus on what is wrong, positive psychology seeks to integrate the fullness of the human experience, which includes both good and bad aspects. Positive psychologists understand and appreciate the limitations associated with seeing the field as merely "happiology."

Positive psychology grows out of robust research on subjective well-being. It has links with humanistic psychology and other avenues of inquiry that emphasize wellness.

One of the core tools we use in the application of positive psychology in Functional Medicine health coaching is the identification of character strengths, the building blocks for health and well-being.

Character Strengths

The VIA Institute on Character was created with a mission to advance the science and practice of character strengths. In 2004, after three years of work by Martin Seligman and Christopher Peterson (also involving 55 renowned scholars and practitioners), Character Strengths and Virtues was published.

The VIA classification offers a common language for discussing what is best in human beings. It provides a framework for us to discuss these positive personality characteristics that are universal to the human experience. Described as essential for a good life, character strengths are the elements of strong and virtuous behaviors. They are qualities that we value in ourselves, our friends, our children, our colleagues, and our leaders. Each person has a unique configuration of the 24 character strengths. They are valued across time, nationalities, and religions.

The VIA classification of character strengths consists of 24 strengths of character nested under six higher-order categories called "virtues." Over three million people from every country in the world have taken the VIA Survey, resulting in the largest database in the world on character strengths. Hundreds of scientific papers have been published in professional journals.

Signature strengths are the core of our identity. They feel authentic and energizing when expressed, as they come naturally to us. They are displayed time and time again throughout our lives and across multiple life domains and situations. Family and friends may note them as fundamental to who we are. Studies link the practice of using signature strengths with greater levels of well-being. For example, the use of signature strengths can be effective in alleviating depression.

In Functional Medicine health coaching, clients are asked to identify and leverage their signature strengths in new ways. In doing so, they access a previously untapped power for creating healing and well-being. Often these strengths are the ones a client takes for granted or discounts as merely "the way they've always been." To the trained Functional Medicine health coach, these strengths stand out as access points for personal growth and positive transformations. By mindfully cultivating one's character strengths, the mental, emotional, and spiritual heart of the Functional Medicine Matrix "lights up" to create a healing response that radiates to all other areas of this interconnected web of physiological systems.

The 6 virtues and 24 character strengths, as identified by the VIA Institute on Character, are the following:

Wisdom and Knowledge (the cognitive strengths)
- Creativity
- Curiosity
- Judgment
- Love of learning
- Perspective

Courage (the emotional strengths)
- Bravery
- Perseverance
- Honesty
- Zest

Humanity (the interpersonal strengths)
- Love
- Kindness
- Social intelligence

Justice (the civic strengths)
- Teamwork
- Fairness
- Leadership

Temperance (the protective strengths)
- Forgiveness
- Humility
- Prudence
- Self-regulation

Transcendence (the spiritual strengths)
- Appreciation of beauty and excellence
- Gratitude
- Hope
- Humor
- Spirituality

Strengths have been found to predict well-being over and above self-esteem and self-efficacy. They have also been linked to increased happiness, work satisfaction, meaning, self-esteem, goal achievement, positive affect, vitality, and lower perceived stress. While character strengths can be systematically and deliberately developed, the starting place for the Functional Medicine health coach is always in noticing and leveraging these 24 character strengths.

How do you grow your character strengths?

- Become aware of your existing character strengths by taking the online VIA survey at www.via.character.org. It will give you a list of the 24 strengths in rank order, from the signature strengths you express the most to the ones you express the least.
- Explore the strengths that interest you, especially your signature strengths — the ones that you apply most naturally in multiple settings and that bring you the most energy. Also, explore the strengths at the bottom of your list. Sometimes there is benefit in investing time to develop a strength that does not come easily to you.
- Take action to use your strengths mindfully as you work toward meeting goals or solving problems.

All change begins with awareness. Many people are not aware of their best qualities, and those that are aware may take their strengths for granted.

How Functional Medicine Health Coaches Use Strengths

In Functional Medicine health coaching, both the coach and the client use their character strengths, primarily their signature strengths — those traits that make us who we are. When we are thriving, we display signature strengths. Through strength-spotting and the application of character strengths, clients can successfully reach their goals and sustain progress in each of the five modifiable lifestyle categories. When they encounter obstacles along the way, they employ character strengths to overcome them and keep going.

The Functional Medicine health coach helps clients become unstuck and move forward by focusing on what is right and strong in them rather than on weaknesses and things that need to be changed. Helping clients identify and use their signature strengths can be the launching pad for helping them make more adaptive and better decisions, including diet and lifestyle choices.

One of the best ways to notice character strengths and express growth involves reflecting on a difficult time in your life as if you were a journalist writing a redemptive narrative. How would a storyteller describe the challenges you faced? What would a good observer see as a turning point in your story? Was there a moment when you re-engaged or found meaning by using a combination of the 24 character strengths? If a journalist were to follow you for a week, what evidence would the journalist see of your strength and resilience? What did you do that demonstrates your growth or expresses your values?

What would family, friends, co-workers, and others who witnessed your journey say to describe how you changed or grew?

Strength-spotting is one of the best activities to help clients engage their strengths. It can be done with any of the 24 strengths, which are often expressed in combinations. There are two levels of strength-spotting: spotting strength in the action of others and spotting strength in your own actions. These levels can occur in any order; however, people commonly report that it's easier to spot strengths in others than in yourself. So, your relationships are a good place to start.

The Functional Medicine health coach might advise clients to enter their next work meeting or family gathering wearing a strength detector — a mindset to look for strengths as they occur. If you spot your co-workers asking a lot of questions, you're noticing their "curiosity" strength. If they're collaborating on projects, you're observing their "teamwork" strength. If someone compliments you, they're displaying their "appreciation of beauty and excellence strength." After you spot the strength, you might name it or tell the person how much you value their strength use.

The Functional Medicine health coach helps clients become aware of their character strengths by asking them to take the VIA survey. They retell the medical story that was created on the Functional Medicine Timeline by adding the strengths history. In the process, they help clients create an alternative narrative that's redemptive and empowering.
For example, if a client describes a history of chronic illness or describes pain, losses, or personal

setbacks, the coach might retell the story by describing the strengths of "hope," "bravery," "perseverance" (not giving up until a healing solution is found), "love of learning" (going online to acquire more knowledge about a particular condition or treatment), or "leadership" (taking control of your health). Other important strengths, including "perspective," "forgiveness," "gratitude," and "spirituality" might emerge when the coach listens mindfully to the story.

By asking questions and sharing observations, Functional Medicine health coaches support clients as they strengths-spot in themselves and others. The coaching conversation may also center around discussing a particular strength and then designing an action plan based on that strength to help the client stick with lifestyle goals.

The following chapters describe lifestyle interventions that are instrumental in healing patterns of chronic illness. In the process of reviewing these interventions, we invite you to observe your relationship to them through the lens of your strengths. If you're supporting someone whose life might greatly benefit from the interventions described, we invite you to highlight their strengths. In so doing, you may help them find access to their internal power and motivation to heal.

Make the Connection: Strengths-Spotting and the Functional Medicine Approach

Heather Aardema, Colorado, USA

Sometimes clients may believe that they haven't made much progress, but then when we start talking, they realize they have. I have met three times now with one woman, and at the last session, I set up the conversation by asking her, "So tell me what went well? How was your week?"

She replied, "Oh, it was a really hard week. I really didn't make much progress." And I said, "Well, remind me — what did we talk about last time?" So she went down the list of what we had discussed during the last session and realized, "Oh, I did that. Oh. Oh, I did that, too." One of her goals was to talk to her boss about a stand-up desk at the office. That was a big deal to her.

I asked, "Have you talked to your boss?"

"Oh, yeah, I did. He said 'Yes.' "

Speaking to her boss meant she was using the "bravery" strength.

As she went down the list, she realized, "Wow, I really thought that I had some struggles, but actually, I did have a lot of wins this week." I suggested the possibility that she was having an emotionally stressful week, causing her to be extra hard on herself. "But now, let's focus on this next week and see how really amazing you can make it."

Daniela Cook, Dubai, United Arab Emirates

I had my children take the VIA survey so I would know their strengths. It was amazing. When I saw my daughter's results, "zest" was number three. That was an "Aha!" moment for me because it helped me see my daughter's love for life. However, that strength only came through when she became gluten-free. It made me realize how impactful nutrition is — not just on physical well-being but also on personality.

Veronica Lim, London, United Kingdom

The things my client said really allowed me to strength-spot with her. When we had our first conversation, she told me she was "all or nothing." That gave me a clue as to the level of perseverance she would have once she made up her mind to do something. I sensed that she would actually stick with her wellness goals.

She was also very honest and had a really great sense of humor. I remember a conversation we had one time when she was complaining about eating healthy and how expensive it was. I said, "Well, what do you think it might cost if you became really sick and someone had to care for you at home?" She just laughed and said, "All right, all right. Let's move on."

Humor was one of the things that really helped the coaching relationship. We were able to tap into that strength when things got a little bit tough from time to time.

For example, sometimes she would say, "Okay, I'm just going to let my hair down this weekend" (meaning she would put less attention on her diet and environmental factors.) We'd chat about how she was going to manage that: Did she want to manage it in the first place, or did she just want to go all out and forget about everything for the weekend? We came up with strategies to help her handle these situations in a way that fit for her.

As I was coaching her about recognizing how her eating patterns in the past led to cravings, her "humility" strength emerged. She said, "You know, it's been really helpful getting to understand about this because, to be honest, I thought I knew it all. But actually, I realize there's so much that I don't know."

As a coach, my top strength is forgiveness. At the end of our sessions, this client shared that she really appreciated that I didn't tell her off for not consistently sticking to the action plan. That was what enabled her to say, "Okay, I can keep with this plan." This was unexpected. I didn't think it would play out that way in terms of someone actually coming back and saying, "Well, actually, I'm glad you weren't beating me up for not doing what I said I would do." Bringing my "forgiveness" strength to the sessions helped her progress.

By helping their clients effectively identify and leverage their strengths, these Functional Medicine health coaches guided their clients to become active champions of their own healing.

Over time, the process of helping clients shift their focus enables them to see solutions where they previously saw symptoms and identify resources where they previously saw roadblocks. We've seen first-hand the cumulative impact this has for clients.

rewrite a different story about themselves and their chronic illness. Instead of seeing themselves as someone who's been "diagnosed with Hashimoto's Disease," they see themselves as someone who is applying the strength of perseverance to "heal a thyroid imbalance."

The distinction in language may seem inconsequential, but to the Functional Medicine health coach, the difference in language connotes a distinction in the client's mind about the location of their power and their life outcomes. This mindset shift underpins and influences the results of all the client's efforts to heal.

Rewriting your story isn't just a matter of semantics. For our coaches and their clients, we've seen that it's often a matter of life and death. As you examine the environmental interventions noted in the following chapters, we invite you to keep in mind two questions:

No matter the diagnosis or symptoms, how would someone accessing his or her strengths make the necessary lifestyle changes that would target the root causes of his or her illness?

How could a coach provide the support needed to enlist one's strengths to change day-to-day behaviors that impact health?

Part 2: The Strategies of Functional Medicine

The following section provides an overview of information about the restorative power of nutrition, exercise, sleep, and relaxation. Many of the Functional Medicine thought-leaders, including FMCA faculty members, have developed protocols in these areas that they have outlined in evidence-based publications, which you can find in the appendix.

Through "Questions a Coach Would Ask," we share with you how Functional Medicine health coaches implement the diet and lifestyle recommendations advocated by Functional Medicine practitioners. These questions are designed to help you start or continue your journey with Functional Medicine.

Ultimately, we invite you to take steps to direct your own healing and trust your innate wisdom. As you read this information, we hope you find deep resonance with the approach. Our appendix section will help you find a Functional Medicine health coach or become one if you believe that this path is right for you.

Chapter 4: Eat and Rebuild

"Let food be thy medicine, medicine be thy food." — Hippocrates

While the possible interventions in Functional Medicine are numerous, the place to start is almost invariably with food. By choosing the right foods and avoiding the wrong ones, it's possible to take back your health. That's the simple message that Functional Medicine health coaches teach their clients.

Dr. Tom O'Bryan, author of The Autoimmune Fix: How to Stop the Hidden Autoimmune Damage That Keeps You Sick, is one of the world's foremost authorities on gluten and autoimmune conditions. Here's how he discovered his path to wellness through food:

"I was not one of those men who always knew he wanted to be a doctor or who was motivated to become one because of a firsthand experience with chronic illness. In fact, I always thought I was a healthy kid. Even though I'm known the world over for my work on autoimmunity and gluten sensitivity, in my early 20s, I was a baker in an organic restaurant in Ann Arbor, Michigan.

Ironically, I used to bake the best bread. People would come from miles around for my unleavened, whole grain, organic bread. I was so hungry all the time when I was younger. I remember I would often take the bread out of the oven, slice off an end piece, spread peanut butter on it, then drizzle honey on it, and lay sliced bananas on top.

I thought I was being so healthy. It was whole wheat bread and organic peanut butter and honey. The bananas were natural. Honey is natural and certainly better than processed sugar. Yet feeding that one hunger craving was probably the worst thing I could have been doing for my health. I was eating a blood sugar time bomb.

I was hungry and tired all the time because of my own chronic low blood sugar, but this snack was flooding my body with the equivalent of four Snickers bars. I would feel great for a while, but the unavoidable crash would happen about an hour later, and I'd be exhausted all over again. I was just trying to live the healthiest life I could, so I kept eating my organic whole wheat bread, not recognizing the damage it was causing."

Food, Inflammation and Chronic Illness

What Dr. O'Bryan didn't know at the time was that the gluten, dairy, and sugar in foods he believed were healthy were contributing to his ill health and fatigue. These are common triggers that set up the entire mechanism of inflammation, one of the main drivers of chronic diseases, including autoimmune conditions. Food isn't just calories. The right amount of the right foods can be more powerful than any medicine, while the wrong amount of the wrong foods leads to harmful consequences — in particular, inflammation.

We associate inflammation with pain, redness, and swelling, the normal physiological responses to a foreign invader. For example, when we have swollen glands or an infected cut, these areas may look red, feel tender to the touch, and cause pain. At FMCA, we teach that an inflammatory response is the body's natural defense mechanism. Cytokines are cells that release chemicals in order to remove the threat. But the inflammation that drives chronic disease is painless and invisible. It's the immune system setting the body on fire to fight off the endless assaults from external dangers, such as potentially harmful foods (processed junk foods, inflammatory fats, gluten, excess sugar), environmental toxins, stress, and internal foes, including harmful bacteria in the gut.

More than half of the immune system resides in our gastrointestinal tract, and when alien substances are detected, this defense system attacks the invaders. It does so by triggering an increase in cytokines, the inflammatory molecules that distinguish between friend and foe. We want them to do their job fighting off infection and destroying cancer cells. But when these inflammatory cytokines get out of control, chronic disease results.

Although the prevailing view of autoimmune disease continues to be that they are inherited genetic conditions involving the immune system suddenly attacking the body, Functional Medicine offers a newer, more plausible explanation. According to Dr. Jeffrey Bland, "Our physiological defense process is in constant communication with how we live, what we eat, and our environment." These factors are continually talking to our immune system, which continually determines whether it is hearing from a friend or foe. Autoimmune diseases, such as rheumatoid arthritis, systemic lupus erythematosus (SLE), multiple sclerosis, Hashimoto's thyroiditis, and many more, arise from an altered immune response.

Autoimmune dysfunction occurs when environmental factors tip the immune system off balance.

Here's how Dr. O'Bryan explains the underlying mechanisms: "Imagine that the human body is a chain of interconnected organs and systems. Whenever you pull on a chain, it will always break at the weakest link. Wherever your weak link is in your body, that's where inflammation will impact, causing symptoms. This weak link might be why you have a vague sense of not feeling well. Perhaps it's weight, perhaps it's memory, perhaps it's your thyroid, joints, or hormones." The weak link in our chains is where we experience illness.

Inflammation-triggered disease patterns account for most chronic illnesses. Dr. O'Bryan goes on to say, "The number one cause of getting sick and eventually dying of some disease is your immune system trying to protect you." When you look at it this way, almost all chronic illnesses are inflammation-based diseases. If putting the fire out is the goal, then not fueling the fire can begin with elimination of foods we know to be inflammatory. Inflammatory and anti-inflammatory foods have been reviewed in Dr. O'Bryan's The Autoimmune Fix, as well as in books by other Functional Medicine practitioners, such as The Autoimmune Solution by Dr. Amy Myers. We also teach these functional nutrition principles at the Functional Medicine Coaching Academy. While we won't go into details here about which specific foods to eat and why, we will review the general guidelines that underpin a Functional Medicine approach to decreasing inflammation and restoring natural function to the body.

Remove the Bad Stuff

The Elimination Diet

The comprehensive elimination diet has proved to be one of the most powerful tools in the Functional Medicine practitioner's tool kit. Studies show that the foods that most commonly cause inflammation include:

- Gluten
- Dairy
- Sugar
- Eggs
- Shellfish
- Corn
- Soy
- Processed meats

These foods are among those eliminated for three weeks and then added back to the diet through a regimented system designed to expose the connection between specific foods and inflammatory symptoms.

Functional Medicine health coaches play a crucial role in educating, supporting, and encouraging clients as they embark on an elimination diet prescribed by their Functional Medicine physician. The number one question a great Functional Medicine health coach will ask is how a client can use his or her signature character strengths to navigate the challenges of removing inflammatory foods from his or her diet.

The foods we consume might be overly refined and processed, filled with chemicals and hormones.

Foods far enough removed from their original plant or animal form have a "shelf life" and need plastic or a box to be sold in your grocery store. These foods are considered "processed." Processed foods pose challenges to our systems because they lack many nutrients available in their original form. These "food-like" substances are so different from the fresh foods our great-grandparents ate that they tax our gastrointestinal tracts and detoxification systems, signal the overproduction of insulin, and stress the adrenal glands. By completing an elimination diet, we can see with clarity the impact processed foods or foods commonly known to be inflammatory have on the system.

The Diet Diary

Before helping clients create a personalized food plan, the first step may be to find out what they're eating regularly. This can be accomplished with the use of a diet diary for one, three, or seven days. A careful review of the diet diary identifies foods that are eaten frequently and extensively and therefore may be at the root of inflammation.

Because it is outside the Functional Medicine health coach's scope of practice to directly recommend eliminating specific foods, completing a food diary can be a great way to help clients become more mindful of what they're consuming regularly. This awareness can help them make the decision on their own to eliminate potentially harmful foods.

Put in the Good Stuff

Eliminating the causes of inflammation leaves a gap in the diet of the client that is best filled with foods that restore optimal cellular function and repair cellular damage caused by inflammation. The foods that do this best from a Functional Medicine perspective are foods that upgrade the quality of macronutrients (proteins, carbohydrates, and fats) and add the under-consumed micronutrients (vitamins, minerals, and phytonutrients [the colorful pigments in plant foods]). We're talking about foods your great-grandmother would have recognized as food: whole, fresh, and preferably home-cooked.

We have been taught that food is fuel for energy. However, recent research demonstrates that food literally communicates with our genes. Information from the specific foods we eat turns genes on and off. This provides the body with instructions on how to control metabolism from moment to moment. Both macronutrients and micronutrients act as powerful neurochemicals. If you want to turn on anti-inflammatory genes, eat a stalk of broccoli. As Michael Pollan, author of Food Rules, states, eat plants, not something made in a plant.

Dr. Dean Ornish demonstrated that after just three months on an intensive diet and lifestyle change program that included plant-based whole foods, over 500 genes that regulate cancer were beneficially affected. The cancer-causing genes were turned off, and the cancer protective genes were turned on.

Functional Medicine visionaries such as Dr. Mark Hyman believe that what we put at the end of our forks every day is the most powerful medicine we can take to correct the root causes of chronic disease. But even with the perfect diet, the combination of depleted soil, long-term storage, transportation of food, genetic alterations of crops, and increased nutritional demands resulting from a toxic environment may make it impossible for most people to get the full complement of vitamins and minerals we need from food alone. A Functional Medicine practitioner can help clients determine their need for nutritional supplements. The coach then becomes the client's ally to figure out a workable plan for incorporating supplements into a daily regimen.

Given all the conflicting data, it's challenging to determine just what constitutes a healthy diet. At FMCA, we clarify this for our students based on the latest research in functional nutrition. This often leads to a breakthrough in their personal health and facilitates recovery for their clients.

What follows is an overview of four core functional nutrition guidelines we use as a springboard to train Functional Medicine health coaches. Numerous studies have corroborated that these four tenets, when followed consistently, can support healing and symptom abatement in inflammatory disease patterns. However, because Functional Medicine is personalized rather than a "one-size-fits-all approach," we acknowledge that what's health-producing for one person may cause an adverse reaction in someone else.

Eat the Rainbow

Colorful food contains phytonutrients, which play critical roles in maintaining long-term health and fighting chronic illness patterns by supporting the body's ability to detoxify. We find that "eating the rainbow" is a dietary habit that is easy to initiate and, therefore, a wonderful first step. Ideally, the coach would suggest that clients fill their plates with greens first and then add other vegetables to obtain "little bits of a lot of color" for a variety of phytonutrients.

A question we suggest our coaches ask is: "How many of these colors can you consume each day?"

- Dark green
- Blue/purple
- Red/pink
- Orange/yellow
- Brown/white

Included in the appendix section of this book is a Phytonutrient Spectrum, a handout that lists common foods associated with each color category and details the health benefits of each pigment. You may want to print this out and place it on your refrigerator or keep it near your wallet when you go to the grocery store to make choosing the rainbow easier.

Eat Lots of Plants and Choose Good-Quality Protein

Plants contain nearly all the vitamins, minerals, antioxidants, phytonutrients, and fiber that we need in our diet. These are essential for keeping the body in balance, including regulating metabolism. In other words, they make the chemical reactions work properly. Functional Medicine health coaches can help clients incorporate more plants in their diets, often making suggestions such as adding one new vegetable to a weekly meal plan.

Just what constitutes good-quality protein? If you eat

animal protein, think about the food the animal consumed as an indication of quality and health for your own body. Look for 100 percent grass-fed rather than grain-fed meat, as the latter has been linked to inflammation. Avoid eating animals that have been given antibiotics or hormones; also avoid by-products of such animals. If a client is interested, the Functional Medicine health coach can provide specific guidelines, such as lists of fish that are low in mercury and other contaminants.

Eat Healthy Fats

Many people fear fat and still believe that low-fat diets are beneficial. The hypothesis that eating too much saturated fat harms your cardiovascular system has been disproved, and many experts now believe it's fine to include healthy dietary sources of cholesterol. Our brains need cholesterol, and hormones are produced from cholesterol. Functional Medicine health coaches play an important role in debunking myths about the dangers of fats through education about the importance of getting enough fat in one's diet. Dr. Mark Hyman's book Eat Fat, Get Thin is a great resource for perplexed clients.

The standard American diet consists of high quantities of inflammatory refined omega-6 oils such as corn, soy, sunflower, and safflower oils. Many are likely deficient in omega-3 fats, found primarily in wild-caught fish and certain seeds and nuts. Omega-3s are vital for healthy brain function and heart health and have many other benefits. We also need omega-9 fats, which can be found in foods such as olive oil and avocados. Here again, the Functional Medicine health coach can step in and educate clients, but only if they request this knowledge. It is not the role of the coach to act as proselytizer for or against particular food choices.

Eat Fermented Foods

The microorganisms that live in our gut play a key role in digestion and have a positive effect in many ways, including boosting immunity and preserving brain health. Fermented or cultured foods such as yogurt, sauerkraut, kimchi (spicy fermented cabbage popular in Korea), and miso (fermented soybean paste) contain probiotic bacteria vital to good health.

The diverse colony of probiotic bacteria living in our gastrointestinal tracts comprises the line of defense in our immune systems. Historically, we've thought of bacteria as a bad thing and created antibiotics to kill bacteria that cause infection. However, researchers discovered that antibiotics not only kill bacteria that cause infection (e.g., e. coli, staphylococcus, etc.) but also destroy the very bacteria meant to protect us. These "good guys" in our gut are also vulnerable to the effects of stress, pesticides in food, and other toxins we consume. Our diets no longer contain the probiotic-rich fermented foods consumed on a regular basis by our ancestors.

Provided that the client expresses interest in experimenting with fermented foods and does not have any medical conditions that may contradict probiotic foods, FMCA coaches teach clients to get their probiotics from these traditional foods to heal the gut and rebuild and repair immune function. In addition, coaches advocate working with a knowledgeable practitioner to determine whether additional probiotic supplementation is advisable.

Eat Mindfully

We can prepare the most nutritionally balanced meal, but if we gulp it down, don't take the time to chew it properly, multi-task while eating, overeat, or eat for reasons other than hunger, we're stressing our system. As a result, digestion becomes impaired.

Clients frequently choose to create goals that center around increasing mindful eating. They may set an intention to chew each morsel of food at least 25 times before swallowing or eliminate pairing eating with watching television, answering emails, or engaging in other distracting activities that promote mindless eating. Others may decide to live by another of Pollan's food rules: Eat at a table; a desk is not a table.

Just as important to consider as what, how, and when we're eating is why we're eating, which may be the most difficult pattern to change. At FMCA, we teach the psychology of eating principles. The foods we choose to eat and the eating habits we adopt can be considered a reflection of who we are: our personalities, our family, our friends, our cultural heritage, and the society in which we live. We're bombarded by messages about what to eat, ranging from well-meaning advice from nutritional experts to slick advertising campaigns from food corporations.

From a young age, foods become associated with emotions. We often eat when we're sad, angry, lonely, or bored, but also when we're happy, content, or in a celebratory mood. We may eat to please others (or not eat to exercise control or rebel). We associate specific foods with holidays and other special occasions. Eating can be a source of pleasure and a social activity that brings great joy and contributes to a sense of belonging. But it can also lead to feelings of guilt and shame.

Functional Medicine health coaches help clients explore their eating choices and patterns. They support individuals as they discover the social, cultural, and emotional connections to food and experiment with adopting new habits. If the client is on board, they provide suggestions for practicing mindful eating.

Questions a Coach Would Ask

Functional Medicine health coaches facilitate a client-centered process. In this approach, coaches ask for permission before making suggestions and always let clients take the lead regarding what foods they want to incorporate into or eliminate from their diets. They may ask clients to pay attention to everything consumed and notice how various foods make them feel. They may help them create a plan for dining out or celebrating a holiday with family or friends.

Questions a trained Functional Medicine health coach might ask to facilitate their client's growth include:

- Do you notice any differences in mental clarity or energy level with certain foods?
- Which foods result in calm and contentment?
- What went well with your food plan this week?

- May I make a suggestion? How about we look at the restaurant menu and discuss possible choices?

While a client may not notice the difference immediately after eating, the positive effects of significant dietary changes will soon become apparent. A coach provides encouragement along the way and reminds clients to call upon the "perseverance" character strength, as the healing process takes time and patience.

Make the Connection: Functional Medicine Approach to Food and Inflammation

Julie Henderson, Arizona, USA

I was bedridden for much of my 30s and early 40s. I lost decades! Married to an internal medicine doctor, I thought there was a pill for every ill, but Western medicine failed me miserably. I went on my own journey to find a different way to treat rheumatoid arthritis other than the typical drugs. I healed my gut with various supplements and eliminated all gluten, dairy, soy, corn, and sugar from my diet. As a result, I overcame severe rheumatoid arthritis!

Lisa Itzcovitch, California, USA

I always followed a healthy diet, but I had to learn how my body was affected by various foods. Even though particular foods were healthy, my body didn't deal with them well. I had to change my eating plan, and I now feel so much better. That, to me, is the motivation. My issues were allergies and asthma. I sought the best specialists but found that they just didn't know what the problem was. "Take some more cortisone cream, inhalers, or steroids," they'd say. When I simply stopped eating nightshades, all my eczema went away, and I haven't used a steroid cream or an inhaler since. That's just a small example.

Heather Aardema, Colorado, USA
Cooking is meditative for me. I love food prepping and planning, and I love knowing that what I'm making for my family members will benefit them and their long-term health.

It's such a gift. I know I'm giving a gift to my family, as well as to myself. What brings me joy is knowing that my kids are not addicted to sugar. They don't eat grains or dairy. I feel like our house is a safe zone. Anything we have in our house the entire family can safely eat.

When my kids go out of the house, they make food decisions for themselves. They determine what they're going to put in their mouths. But in our home, we have an abundance of fruits and vegetables. We do the color wheel.

Marian Condon, Pennsylvania, USA
I have learned to always have good food in the car. If I let myself get really hungry while in front of a store with something enticing inside, I might buy it, regardless of whether or not it would hurt me. My love affair with sweets is not over, but it's controllable now. As long as I make sure I'm not dehydrated or super hungry, I can walk past almost anything without really even looking twice.

I feel that I have been freed from prison. I used to be a slave to sugar. When I say that to people, they think I'm exaggerating; people who haven't been there don't understand it. I really was enslaved by sugar, and now I am free.

Jesse Proctor, North Carolina, USA
I think one of the most profound and surprising shifts in my health came from diet. I have been an organic farmer for five years, and the quality of my food has been good, but FMCA introduced me to very specific diets for more specific problems. I tried many of the functional nutrition food plans developed by IFM to see how they would affect my body. These food plans were truly life-changing for me. When you find the right relationship with food, the results can be really positive. I discovered that the wrong diet versus the right diet can be the difference between dealing with severe inhibitors (such as not being able to get out of bed, severe neuropathy, and confusion) and being able to climb a mountain.

Daniela Cook, Dubai, United Arab Emirates
On a daily basis, I try to make sure the kids eat the rainbow, so there are always different colors on their plate. They know that half their plate has to be vegetables, no matter what shape or size, and that they have to eat them. We go by the 80-20 rule, so as long as they're good 80 percent of the time, I'm prepared to close an eye the other 20 percent, although I always exclude gluten for my daughters. My son is a full-blown teenager; there's no way he's going to listen to me telling him not to eat sweets. However, I heard him tell his friends the other day that eating sugar would depress his immune system. So I know the information is getting in there.

Each of these stories showcases the power of starting where you are with what works for you and your family. Knowing both your strengths and your triggers can support you on the path toward sustainable dietary change, but it all starts with awareness.

At the Functional Medicine Coaching Academy, we support and encourage our students to embark on their own healing journey through food as medicine by "taking out the bad stuff" and "putting in the good stuff" and exploring the meaning of food in their lives.

We also train our coaches to respect the pace of a client's transformation. This means emphasizing that if a client shows up for coaching, he or she already won half the battle, choosing to get well and believe that wellness is possible personally and for his or her family. By bringing mindfulness, hope, and compassion to each coaching session, the coach keeps the client in the game. The coach acts as a personal cheerleader, providing education as needed and letting the client be the guide that leads the way.

Chapter 5: Sleep and Relax

"Stress is harmful, except when it's not. Stress increases the risk of heart problems, except when people regularly give back to their communities. Stress increases the risk of dying, except when people have a sense of purpose. Stress increases the risk of depression, except when people see a benefit in their struggles. Stress is paralyzing, except when people perceive themselves as capable. Stress is debilitating, except when it helps you perform. Stress makes people selfish, except when it makes them altruistic." — Dr. Kelly McGonigal, clinical psychologist; author, The Upside of Stress

Address Stress

Functional Medicine health coaching helps clients become better at living with stress. Rather than attempting to reduce or avoid stress, embracing stress may help people heal, even in very difficult situations. Embracing stress changes how we think about ourselves and what we think we can handle. Focusing on the upside of stress transforms how we experience it, both physically and emotionally.

At FMCA, we identify five core ways to address stress:

- Reframe stress. Find a way to see the contribution stress makes instead of the toll it takes.
- Connect with others. Experience the joys of social connection to reset the central nervous system.

- Get ample rest. Harness the power of sleep for detoxification and repair.
- Practice relaxation techniques. Intentionally manage the nervous system's response to daily and ongoing stress through meditation, breathing, and mindfulness.
- Prioritize positivity. Rather than experiencing the angst of a stressful situation, this action, rooted in positive psychology, facilitates positive health changes.

Reframe Stress

Conventional wisdom holds that stress is bad and must be reduced or managed. However, research evidence shows that it's the combination of stress and the belief that stress is harmful that's dangerous. As a result, we're challenging how we think about stress. Evidence suggests that stress can make one smarter, stronger, and more successful. It can promote growth and inspire courage and compassion.

Kelly McGonigal, health psychologist and author of The Upside of Stress, defines stress as what arises when something you care about is at stake. In other words, stress and meaning are linked. You cannot create a meaningful life without experiencing some stress.

The Functional Medicine model of health coaching incorporates this new interpretation of stress and teaches coaches to help clients reframe and reinterpret stress. They do so by creating a redemptive narrative and drawing upon character strengths.

To facilitate the reframing of stress, Functional Medicine health coaches explore how adversity makes one stronger. For example, a coach could prompt a client to identify a period of significant personal growth in his or her life — a turning point that led to positive changes or a new direction or purpose. Next, the coach might ask if the client would also describe this time as stressful. Through questioning, the coach helps the client reframe stress and change his or her interpretation of stress concerning current circumstances. This allows the client a much-needed emotional and mental reprieve that can foster continued recovery once he or she is no longer "stressed" about a health challenge.

Celebrating the positive changes as we grow from difficult experiences can be supported through coaching. The good that comes from challenging experiences is not from the stressful or traumatic event itself, but from the strengths that are awakened by adversity and by the capacity to transform suffering into meaning. Part of embracing stress involves trusting this capacity, even when the pain is fresh and the future is uncertain.

Trauma or loss generates tremendous suffering, but, at the same time, these can inspire positive change. This phenomenon is referred to as post-traumatic growth. The Posttraumatic Growth Research Group defines this phenomenon as "positive change experienced as a result of the struggle with a major life crisis or a traumatic event."

Survivors of almost every imaginable kind of physical and psychological trauma report this effect. It has been documented in children and adults in various cultures and countries around the globe. Survivors of trauma who experience post-traumatic growth might say the following: "I have a greater sense of closeness with and compassion for others." "I'm stronger than I thought I was." "I have a greater appreciation for the value of my own life." "I have a stronger religious faith." "I established a new path for my life."

Those who experience post-traumatic growth tell a redemptive story. By calling upon character strengths, and with the alliance of a Functional Medicine health coach, clients can find post-traumatic growth.

Connect with Others

One of the best ways to transform stress is by utilizing the power of social connection. When overwhelmed by stress, one can find hope by connecting rather than escaping. The sense of suffering in isolation is one of the biggest barriers to transforming stress.

Going further and helping others is also an effective way to transform stress. When we feel alone and disconnected, it may be difficult to see any good in the current struggle. While invisibility often goes hand-in-hand with chronic illnesses, online groups such as https://www.patientslikeme.com are taking the isolation out of healing.

Functional Medicine health coaches might suggest that clients leverage their strengths to facilitate social connection, whether online or offline. For example, for clients whose strength is forgiveness, coaches may suggest processes for forgiveness to restore harmony and alleviate stress in the clients' relationships.

Get Ample Rest and Relaxation

According to Functional Medicine physician Dr. Mark Menolascino, coaches can really shine in a Functional Medicine practice by helping clients with sleep. Often, the key to viewing stress differently is a good night's rest. To have the physical and psychological energy to transform stress, one needs to prioritize rest and relaxation.

Sleep tends to be undervalued in contemporary society. We tend to believe a common myth that we can teach ourselves to get by on less sleep and not experience problems. That is false. The adult human brain requires at least seven hours of sleep per night to function at its best. Getting enough sleep and getting quality sleep may be the keys to health. One of the most restorative things we can do for deeply stressful situations is get ample sleep.

Changing sleep habits requires motivation. A Functional Medicine coach can increase a client's motivation by reviewing why better sleep habits have value. In The Healing Power of Sleep: A Guide to Healthy and Refreshing Sleep Skills, Dr. Lynn Johnson states that individuals who get a sufficient amount of sleep learn new skills better. Dreaming is the time in which one symbolically practices these new skills.

When we get at least seven hours of sleep each night, we're more likely to resist infections, including colds and the flu. That's because ample sleep promotes a healthier immune system. Sleep deprivation contributes to blood sugar dysregulation, obesity, and difficulty losing weight. People who miss sleep tend to eat more, particularly foods high in sugar, to make up for the lack of energy they experience.

Our bodies repair and restore themselves during sleep. Crucial detoxification processes take place as well. Furthermore, the parasympathetic branch of the autonomic nervous system associated with the relaxation response is restored with sleep. That's why we feel relaxed after a good night's rest.

We can improve sleep through learning and practicing sleep hygiene — those habits that foster better sleep. Can we learn better sleep hygiene? Experts agree that a change in behavior is the best treatment for sleep. In other words, sleep is nothing but a set of habits, and we can change our habits. Functional Medicine health coaches support and guide clients as they establish better sleep hygiene.

According to Dr. Menolascino, research shows our bodies need a predictable schedule. Coaches encourage clients to experiment with going to bed at approximately the same time each night and awakening at the same time each morning. They can follow up with questions such as "What did you notice when you stuck with this routine?" A coach might suggest that a client keep a sleep diary. Can the client look for nights when he or she slept unusually well? What was different or unique about those days?

While we have an important need for nighttime sleep, there's also emerging evidence about the importance of daytime rest and how the two are connected. A restful state throughout the day seems to be just as important as the rest that takes place during the night.

Functional Medicine health coaches can help clients train their brains to quiet down. This may take the form of some type of meditation or relaxation technique. However, the Functional Medicine health coach approach mandates that coaches don't impose their beliefs on clients. What's relaxing to one person may be stress-producing to someone else. Functional Medicine health coaches ask questions such as "What brings you joy?" "What activities do you find relaxing?" "What do you think about learning meditation?"

Prioritize Positivity

Dr. Barbara Fredrickson, a world-renowned positive psychology researcher, advocates "prioritizing positivity" to help one feel relaxed and renewed each day. Prioritizing positivity is a proactive way of arranging your day so you have experiences that you know are very likely to make you experience positive emotions. Fredrickson prioritizes positivity for herself by scheduling an outdoor walk each morning. She puts in her earbuds and engages in a phone conversation with her sister, who is also walking but far away in another state. Although they live far apart, they look forward to "nature bathing" together.

According to Fredrickson, at one level, everyone values happiness and wants to be happy. But people differ in how they plan their days. She believes that's "where the rubber meets the road." Many of us plan each day solely around achievement. "I have to get this done." "I have to accomplish this." Daily activities are often structured around "should" and "need to" and not around doing things that will generate positive emotions.

Functional Medicine health coaches can play a major role in guiding clients to look at what they're doing to prioritize rest and relaxation. They may ask, "How are you setting aside time to relax, restore, and find peace and calm?" "What will you do each day to prioritize positivity?"

We invite you to prioritize positivity in your life. If this is the only step you take, it's the step that will reap the biggest rewards.

Questions a Coach Would Ask

Because Functional Medicine health coaching is client-centered, it's up to the client to determine how he or she wants to prioritize positivity and engage in a relaxing activity. A dictator coach would tell a client to take a yoga class, learn to meditate, or practice deep breathing for a prescribed number of minutes per day. However, as we mentioned earlier, the coach who utilizes the Functional Medicine approach recognizes that what's relaxing or pleasurable for one person may trigger stress for someone else.

Here are some questions a coach might ask to support a client in this area:

- How are you setting aside time to relax, restore, and find peace and calm?
- May I offer a suggestion? What do you think about starting a meditation practice?
- How do you think you can use your strength of "X" to help you get more sleep and relaxation?
- What kind of activity leaves you feeling refreshed and restored?

- What kind of support do you feel you need to help you get the right kind of sleep?
- If you were to fit more relaxation and sleep into your schedule, how would you do that?

Asking these questions of yourself and offering them to clients can provide the spark for the mind to create solutions where there were previously challenges. These are the kinds of questions that led to transformative experiences for our students and clients in the stories that follow.

Make the Connection: Address Stress through a Functional Medicine Approach

Terra Santos, Kentucky, USA
I had five children, and at the time, I was homeschooling. We were living in toxic mold, so we ended up having to move and leave our things behind. It was a nightmare. More than anything, I found myself struggling with guilt over the choices I made to get myself healthy. I took the bad foods out of my diet because that change didn't significantly impact my day-to-day interactions. But when it came to self-care, I could very easily say, "I've got five kids. When do I have time to do that?"

I remember telling my coach how much I enjoyed yoga, but I just couldn't fit it into my day. She helped me break apart what I was doing step-by-step so I could see what was working for me and what I enjoyed. I started going to the YMCA two to three days per week. I felt guilty putting the kids in childcare because I was coming from a homeschooling perspective. I wasn't used to sending them off to school.

My oldest was nine, and my youngest was one. I remember telling my coach, "I feel guilty. The younger kids like it, but the older kids hate it. They feel like babies." She very gently encouraged me to think about how much better of a mom and a person I could be when I was able to take that time for myself.

The YMCA offered three hours of childcare, and I would take 55 minutes for my class and then rush to get everybody and head out because I felt guilty. To this day, as often as possible, I take the full three hours, and that's how I got a lot of my coursework done for FMCA. I would go to a class and do a lot of my coursework during that time. It was good for me, and I needed to do it. It also turned out to be good for my kids.

My coach gave me lots of those little insights that encouraged me to see how I could take care of myself, how I could be a better mom, wife, and friend, etc. Again, I knew all these things, but very practically, I just didn't know how to apply them. She was so patient in listening to me and debunking some of the "mess in my head."

Lawrence Robbins, Hong Kong, China
Every morning, my wife and I get up early. We don't sleep in and wait until the last moment, leaving ourselves only 20 minutes to get up, get a shower, get dressed, and get out the door. We really enjoy having that relaxing time. I have my big mug of coffee and like to take the time to sit down and enjoy this experience and not rush. I think that's one of the keys

to reducing stress levels and just remaining calm in general.

Jesse Proctor, North Carolina, USA
I have found that it's necessary and important to give myself permission to set a lot of boundaries in this healing process. So many of us know that we need enough sleep and do well with eight hours. We know that feeling less stressed helps us be physically healthier. We know these things, and still it can be so hard to give ourselves permission to make sure we prioritize these things.

It's only because I've been so sick that self-care is my only option. If I want to get out of bed, function, have a job, have relationships, go hiking, go kayaking, etc., I simply have to create these boundaries for myself. My priority has to be sleeping enough, eating the right things, and making sure I don't have any seriously toxic relationships in my life.

Heather Shover, Texas, USA
I'd say the biggest impact for me has been meditation and breathing techniques. After I physically healed, I had so much energy. It was suddenly like, "Oh, wow." I experienced a heightened sense of awareness. A sense of life's purpose came to me that I had never had before.

I meditate in the morning. I get up around six o'clock, before the household gets up, and I do my breathing and some meditation prayer. I end with ten Yoga Sun Salutations. Then I feel like I'm ready for the day.

I've been doing meditation practice for just about a year now. It's a lot of guided visualizations. I picture myself as a tree with roots in the earth and branches. Because I've done this visualization over and over, it now doesn't take long to imagine growing my roots and branches.

When I started, I meditated for twenty minutes. Now even two minutes makes a big difference. I imagine a deep grounding and become aware that I'm pulling the resources from the earth — from the universe — and I'm calm.

———

The Functional Medicine health coach approach to addressing stress has everything to do with listening to clients' stories, encouraging post-traumatic growth, and helping clients use character strengths to build resiliency as they start the healing journey.

In each of these stories, you may have noticed that time was a recurring challenge. Making time, feeling guilty about how much time is necessary, creating boundaries around time, and committing to the time to create ritual and routine are common challenges for all of us. Functional Medicine health coaches provide support as clients negotiate time challenges in a way that leaves them empowered as opposed to energetically drained by "one more thing."

We've repeatedly seen that immersion in the five core ways to address stress outlined in this chapter creates a significant transformation in the lives of the coaches that graduate from FMCA. Students enroll in FMCA out of a desire to become a Functional Medicine Certified Health Coach. However, immersion in Functional Medicine, positive psychology, and mind-body medicine curriculum, combined with the personal exploration exercises that they engage in, leads to unintended consequences. FMCA graduates report that they radically transform their relationship to stress through reframing it, connecting with others, getting ample rest, practicing relaxation techniques, and prioritizing positivity. These practices become the foundation for work with clients. They coach effectively, not just because they were trained to do so, but because they implement these principles in their own lives.

Chapter 6: Change Your Mind to Move Your Body

"Our bodies are our gardens, to which our wills are gardeners." — William Shakespeare

Everyone has heard the adage that exercise is the best medicine. Lack of exercise creates low-grade inflammation, whereas regular exercise can dramatically reduce inflammation. Important for both physical and mental health, exercise may be critical for the prevention and even the reversal of chronic disease.

In an ideal world, we'd all have a workout routine that incorporates activities to build endurance, strength, and flexibility. We've heard about the many benefits of exercise, yet most Americans struggle to get enough physical movement in any form. Why can't we "just do it?"

An emphasis on the physical effects of exercise may be partly to blame for our apathy about physical activity. Physicians frequently tell patients to engage in a workout routine to lose weight, lower cholesterol, or prevent chronic illness. But this approach may be a recipe for failure. Demonstrable physical results are not always immediately apparent. In addition, when an authority figure tells us we should be doing something, that directive may create a stress response within us, causing us not to comply.

The mood boost that exercise creates, on the other hand, offers near-instant gratification. Functional Medicine health coaches encourage clients to tune in to their mental state after exercise. Suppose someone was feeling down or lethargic and then went outside for a walk. A question a coach might ask is this: "On a scale of one to ten, with one being completely miserable and ten being fantastic — on top of the world — how would you rate how you felt before the walk and afterward?"

At the Functional Medicine Coaching Academy, we recognize that to reap the benefits of exercise, individuals must follow plans that are personalized to fit their needs and preferences. Most importantly, each person's choice of exercise must elicit positive emotions, and the participant needs to believe that the activity is beneficial. As experts in behavior change, Functional Medicine health coaches are in a unique position to help people get off the couch and become motivated to exercise.

In this chapter, rather than explore the positive impact exercise can have, we discuss the mindset required to commit to and sustain a regular exercise routine. The difference between carving out the time to exercise and making excuses for not engaging in physical activity lies in one's mental attitude. Employing a positive psychology approach, Functional Medicine health coaches partner with clients to access their character strengths and increase their motivation to get moving.

Accountability can be one effective aspect of the coach-client relationship that increases commitment to an exercise plan. According to Ruth Wolever, a leader in the field of health coaching, "When we tell another person we're going to do something, and know we have to report back to them, we'll exert

additional effort to make sure we follow through."
Evidence suggests that the support a coach provides
can make it more likely for individuals to stay
motivated and sustain behavior change.

Beginning with baby steps has been shown to be an
effective way to initiate a movement plan. Something
as simple as "Today I will walk around the block for 10
minutes after I finish answering emails" may be a
viable starting place. With this initial goal established,
the client reports back to the coach about the
experience during the next session and creates a new
goal, perhaps extending the walk to 15 minutes.

Positive Emotions Matter

Negative thinking about exercise can cancel out the
positive benefits of exercise in more ways than one.
For example, if it's just another "to do" on your list,
both the mental and physical health benefits may be
negated. Exercise may only have benefits if we're
engaging in an activity that we want to do. If the
activity is so far out of our comfort zone that it brings
up traumatic memories or elicits excessive negative
internal dialogue, we, as advocates for optimal health,
must consider this: Is it really helping? For further
consideration, how many times have we started an
exercise program or joined a gym with the best of
intentions, only to drop out or discontinue because we
had no enthusiasm or other positive emotions to drive
our commitment?

According to Dr. Barbara Fredrickson, positive
emotions increase when people are active. However,
when people work at a very intense, vigorous level,
their positive emotions decrease. She suggests

staying active to the level that positive emotions are maximized, but as soon as the positive emotions start to decline because the exertion is too intense, back off to keep the positive emotions. "Adjust the behavior to keep the positive emotions in the sweet spot. By doing so, we harness the way positive emotions work to get us automatically thinking about that activity . . . When we enjoy an activity, when we're not doing that activity, we're much more likely to have spontaneous thoughts popping into our mind about that activity that are pleasant. The more we have those spontaneous thoughts just pop into mind about that activity, the more we engage in that activity in the coming week."

Dr. Fredrickson believes that when positive emotions are associated with an activity, our unconscious minds send this idea of "I want to practice yoga today" or "I want to get out and take a walk." These spontaneous thoughts steer us to want to do that activity more often. But when we don't enjoy an activity, we don't have those automatic thoughts that direct us toward the life-saving benefits of exercise.

By engineering an activity to maximize the positive emotions, we set up these unconscious motivational streams in a way that makes it easy and natural to pursue the behavior rather than difficult, requiring a lot of willpower. Fredrickson likens this process to what happens when we fall in love.

When we fall in love with someone, that person is always on our minds. We constantly think about and want to be with him or her. When working with clients on exercise goals, the Functional Medicine health coach wants to help them engineer falling in love with an activity so it's always on their minds — something they want to do because positive emotions are created. Rather than nagging you as something you think you should do or that someone else is ordering you to do, exercise can become a favorite passion or favorite activity.

Beliefs about Exercise Matter

In a fascinating study, Alia Crum recruited housekeepers at hotels for research on how beliefs affect weight and height. Housekeeping is strenuous work. As exercise, it's on par with weight lifting or walking at a brisk pace. However, two-thirds of the housekeepers in the study believed they weren't exercising regularly. One-third said they didn't exercise at all. Their bodies reflected this perception. The housekeepers' weight-to-hip ratio, blood pressure, and total body weight were exactly what you would expect to find if they were truly sedentary.

Crum hypothesized that when two outcomes are possible — in this case, the health benefits of exercise or the strain of physical labor — a person's expectations influence which outcome is more likely. To influence the expectations of the housekeepers in the study, Crum designed a poster that described how housekeeping qualified as exercise. Lifting mattresses, picking towels off the floor, pushing heavily loaded carts, and vacuuming require strength and stamina. The poster even included the calories burned while doing each activity.

Housekeepers in other hotels acted as the control group. They were not informed that their work qualified as exercise but received information about the importance of physical exercise for health.

Surprisingly, when Crum looked at the results, those who had been told that their work was exercise lost weight and body fat. Their blood pressure was lower. They even liked their jobs more. They had not made any changes in their behavior outside work. The only thing that changed was their perception of themselves as exercisers. The housekeepers in the control group showed none of these improvements.

The housekeepers' perception of their work as healthy exercise transformed its effect on their bodies. In other words, the effect we expect is the outcome we get.

Questions a Coach Would Ask

We teach Functional Medicine health coaches to explore the client's exercise history, desires, and enjoyments. Through active listening, the coach picks up on clues about the right kind of exercise for the client and, more importantly, the right approach for adding more of it to the client's life. Try these questions on yourself to get a sense of your own relationship to exercise and see what you discover:

- What are your early memories of physical education, team sports, and exercise?
- What are your current feelings about your relationship to exercise?
- What strengths can be applied to starting and sustaining an exercise program? What challenges exist?
- When did you feel better after exercising than before you began? What activity were you engaged in?
- What types of movement bring you joy?
- Do you prefer exercising alone or with a buddy?
- Would you like to explore group classes?
- Do you become bored with one activity and want to try mixing things up?

Make the Connection: The Mindset for Movement

Sharon Falchuk, Massachusetts, USA
Sometimes illness is your greatest teacher; it definitely has been for me. I used to push myself in many ways. I used to try to make myself run and

engage in a strenuous exercise routine. Then I got sick and couldn't exercise at all.

I fell in love with yoga, tai chi, and qigong. Even though it didn't feel like I was engaging in exercise, I decided to change my mindset. I previously thought, "You have to push yourself really hard to be fit." That's false. I learned that pushing myself really hard with exercise wasn't good, mentally or physically.

I know how difficult it can be to exercise while in pain, and I ask clients if they can start out by just pumping their feet in bed. Literally, if that's all you can do, do it. When people tell me, "I can't exercise because I'm in too much pain," I reply, "Okay, you can sit there and roll your wrists or pump your feet."

Marian Condon, Pennsylvania, USA

I felt helpless to control my addiction to sugar. It seemed like food was the best thing in my life. Then I fell in love with ballroom dancing. I mean head-over-heels in love. I realized that I had something in my life that was even more fun than food.

I made new friends at the studio who were more fit. They were thinner because they were into movement. I gradually distanced myself from my eating buddies. I still hang out with them occasionally, but not anywhere near as often. I decided, "Boy, I need to lose this weight so I can dance better." It gave me a tremendous amount of motivation.

Dancing is helpful to me in so many ways. It's even going to help me with clients because I know what it felt like to be desperate, and now I know the joy of movement.

Donna Ott, Pennsylvania, USA

The little boy I coached was living with severe global delays from autism and was under conventional care, with no access to a Functional Medicine doctor.

Coaching kids is parent- and child-focused. Rather than developing a treatment plan, I empowered the parents to develop goals. I encouraged them to trust their wisdom, telling them that they will know better than anyone else how their child responds to the interventions being initiated.

I gently guided the family in transforming many lifestyle factors. We adjusted the cleaning products they used and provided the Environmental Working Group as a resource. The boy's mom became interested in changing his diet to include bone broth and organic foods. She later tried gluten-free and began incorporating a greater diversity of phytonutrients. Regarding his sleep hygiene and relaxation, I encouraged the use of essential oils in a diffuser as well as relaxation techniques for stress management.

My client and his parents are amazing! They were completely devoted to helping him walk, despite the fact that he could barely sit and the pediatrician thought this goal was unrealistic. However, early intervention research supports the parents' objectives, so I supported them in their wish to see their child walk. Parents know their child better than any of us, and I simply encouraged them.

The family was brave and persistent in helping their child learn to walk. They showed an astounding amount of hope, courage, and perseverance. His walking initially seemed reflexive, as he had very poor motor control. They walked him a lot, all day, every day. Physically, it was demanding. It was a beautiful, almost magical sight the day they showed me that he could take two steps between them. He could sit for about 30 seconds, but he took those steps. They were so happy, and so was I.

They continued to constantly practice. He gradually took more and more steps, and they were not afraid to let him try. We all realized that he had both an idea of what he wanted to do — which direction he wanted to walk in — as well as some perception of danger. Naturally he fell, but they helped him back up. Gradually, he walked across their living room and kitchen. He learned to turn, and then to walk outside, including up and down curbs.

At Thanksgiving, I watched him walk up steps with his father holding his hand, and the thought of him a year ago, unable to sit and stuck in repetitive rocking movements much of the time, went through my mind. I felt profound gratitude and joy for this family who was seeing their child progress and develop new skills.

———

Anywhere you look on the Internet or in bookstores, you can find blogs, magazines, and books touting a million reasons to exercise, a million more reasons why people don't, and an endless array of fitness plans of every shape and size. But coming from a strengths perspective, we committed to answering this question: What do people need to start and commit to exercise? What actually works?

People make time for and do what feels good. They avoid what feels bad. It's that simple.

By finding ways for clients to feel good before and during exercise, Functional Medicine health coaches ensure clients have a clear path toward continuing to exercise.

Part 3: Is Functional Medicine Health Coaching Right for You?

In Parts 1 and 2, you were introduced to Functional Medicine and the Functional Medicine health coach. We hope you saw the power of Functional Medicine health coaching through our students and their clients.

In this section, we invite you to take a deeper look at the impact that client-centered Functional Medicine health coaching has on people's lives. We invite you to explore what gives you the greatest meaning and purpose in your own life.

If you have a calling to serve in a new way — a way that makes room for clients' stories and makes sense of seemingly disparate symptoms while trusting the client, not just the physician, to have the answers — then working as a Functional Medicine health coach may be right for you.

Chapter 7: How to Use Client-Centered Coaching

"In my early professional years, I was asking the question: How can I treat, or cure, or change this person? Now I would phrase the question in this way: How can I provide a relationship which this person may use for his own personal growth?" — Carl R. Rogers, psychotherapist, author

In *The Patient Will See You Now*, Eric Topol writes about a revolution in healthcare powered by widespread access to information and personalized medicine. He believes that we're reaching a time in which each person will have access to all his or her own medical data due to the power of technology. This will create a power shift that will put the individual at center stage and the doctor in a satellite support role. Topol predicts that the adage "The doctor will see you now," which implies that power lives with the doctor, will no longer be true. The relationship may be radically altered. Patients will experience greater power of choice regarding their healthcare options.

We see the rapid growth of client-centered health coaching occurring within this larger movement of patient empowerment. As patients increasingly gain access to the same information doctors have, their ability to ask educated questions increases. So, too, does their ability to advocate for and decline care as they see fit. The coaching relationship can further fuel this reclamation of personal power.

According to Dr. Michael Arloski, the role of the health coach may be misperceived by the public and by many healthcare professionals. Often a client is referred to a health coach because the physician believes the client needs to change his or her diet or begin an exercise program. Implicit in the referral is the expectation that the coach will carry out the doctor's orders. However, a client-centered approach implies that goals are created by the client, not dictated by the wishes of the provider or the coach. Rather than incorporating the diet or exercise goals desired by the referring practitioner, change plans might center on finding meaning, working less, or improving social connections as a method of producing viable and sustainable health results.

When a Functional Medicine health coach co-creates wellness goals with a client, the coach evolves from the agenda the client sets. The coach may think the client needs to eat, rest, or exercise differently to attain the desired results. However, the coach always trusts in the client's wisdom and takes direction from him or her. The coach trusts that the client truly wants to get well and is doing his or her best to get there. Although the coach might challenge the client to accomplish more or guide him or her to attempt less, a client-centered approach involves avoiding playing the expert role and letting the agenda and timetable for change come from the client at all times.

In client-centered psychotherapy, developed by Carl Rogers, the therapist has no predetermined agenda but stays with the client and goes where he or she leads.

Applying the same model, Functional Medicine health coaching results in real, sustainable growth. A collaborative relationship depends on the health coach recognizing and acknowledging the client's experience. As opposed to the expert, the coach invites the client to be a whole individual responsible for his or her own choices. Rather than saying "I can help you," the client-centered health coach asks, "How are you hoping I can help you? What kind of support are you looking for?"

When Functional Medicine health coaches work for a medical practitioner, an insurance company, or a corporate wellness program, they may be charged with "getting people to change their habits." But unless they use a client-centered approach, these changes may not happen. When clients are dictated and lectured to, they may feel as if they're being judged or scolded. Their resistance may take the form of non-compliance or non-attendance.

At the Functional Medicine Coaching Academy, we strongly believe in a client-centered approach to coaching. Four key features produce increased client engagement and commitment:

- Establishing rapport
- Using open-ended inquiry
- Becoming an ally
- Creating a meaningful connection

Establish Rapport

Being in rapport means having the ability to enter another person's model of the world, communicating that we truly understand that world in a congruent way. More than simply understanding the client's experience, establishing rapport involves ensuring the client *feels* understood in his or her experience of our understanding.

Perception of being understood must be established. It's critical for engaging someone's trust and functions as the launching pad for actively leveraging the power of the coaching relationship. Essential for getting along with others, building rapport occurs unconsciously throughout our lives whenever we connect meaningfully with others.

Consider one example of rapport in action: the behavior of high school students who are with their friends. Behavioral mirroring (adopting the same ways of speaking, dressing, and behaving), offers of verbal validation, mutual curiosity, and more are common patterns of unconscious rapport-building among high school peers. These patterns can also be selectively employed to establish rapport in a coaching relationship. Ultimately, building rapport consists of creating safety and comfort that act as a permission slip for the other person to be his or her unique self. Consciously building rapport sends the nonverbal message, "You're not alone. You're safe with me because I'm like you, too."

To elicit and understand each client's story, to help people make changes that are beneficial, and to create coaching partnerships, we develop rapport with clients so they feel safe enough to risk change.

Use Open-Ended Inquiry

As opposed to expecting correct or incorrect responses to questions, open-ended inquiry involves establishing dialogue by asking questions to which the answers are anything but "Yes" or "No." These questions or conversation starters typically start with "What," "How/How come," "Tell me about," or "Describe." Through open-ended inquiry, clients reflect on thoughts and feelings. They share their unique perceptions and generate their own solutions.

Closed-ended inquiries usually have single-word or "correct" answers. To answer these questions, clients do not need to provide insight into their experiences. These questions, which can be answered by a simple "Yes" or "No," tend to deal in the realm of facts more than thoughts and feelings and may close off conversations.

Become an Ally

In client-centered coaching, the coach takes the client's side as a way of facilitating the best possible outcome, no matter what happens — no matter what the client does or doesn't do. Coaches who act as a genuine ally choose to see each clients' choices as purposeful. In instances where the coach as ally doesn't understand choices that his or her client made, the coach employs open-ended inquiry to look for strengths and elicit the client's intended positive outcome. In an alliance, the client knows that the coach is a staunch supporter and will remain by his or her side, no matter what choices he or she decides to make. As a result, the client typically remains open to opportunities to try new tactics, particularly when his or her choices haven't yielded the desired results.

Dr. Arloski writes, "When we accept a client as an ally, we stick beside them, not above them, and work at the development of trust. We are open to more closeness than before. We are not sitting in clinical judgment. The client has the answers. The coach has the questions. Coaches engage in a process to help clients find their own answers that they really do have within themselves. We don't motivate anyone. We help them find the motivation they have within themselves."

"Alliance" implies maintaining unconditional positive regard for clients. This concept derives from humanistic psychotherapy and has been defined as the act of seeing another person as whole and worthy, regardless of his or her behavioral choices. We accept clients as they are, not as we wish them to be. By doing so, we refrain from judgment and are perceived as being "on their side."

Create a Meaningful Connection

Through the process of establishing rapport, showing genuine interest by asking open-ended questions, and demonstrating alliance, the Functional Medicine health coach recognizes the client's existence as a valuable part of the whole, and thus the coach's own life. In a client-centered relationship, coaches act as both the teacher and the student — the leader and the follower. Coaches often acknowledge that clients help them learn and grow. In other words, both the coach and the client benefit from the high-quality, meaningful connection that their relationship provides.

Understanding that we're here because we're needed is a resource-rich way of approaching relationships. We encourage clients to adopt this mentality as a way of fueling their wellness journey. This realization can break down isolation and create a sense of belonging for clients. We know from recent research that social bonds can change the course of chronic illness. A sense of belonging and positive connections to others can help people re-establish wellness in their lives. Clients can create stronger ties with family and friends and even connect with strangers or acquaintances by establishing positive short-term interactions.

During a high-quality connection, each person is tuned in to the other and both reciprocate positive regard and care. As a result, both people feel valued. Close personal relationships with family and friends and high-quality coaching connections have an important feature in common — both require us to focus on others and see them as needed and important.

According to Dr. Barbara Fredrickson, helping people develop a lens and an appreciation for the small, everyday sources of positive emotion tied to belonging can be especially helpful. At the end of every day at her research lab, she asks people to reflect on the degree to which they felt connected with others that day. They're instructed to think of their three longest social interactions and rate how in tune they felt with the people they spent time with. She has found that over the course of several weeks, this regular habit of reflecting on connection not only raises positive emotions day in and day out but also improves objective markers of physical health.

Improvement in cardiac vagal tone or heart rate variability has been demonstrated with this simple intervention of reflecting on connection. Fredrickson believes that seeing all interactions as sources of potential positivity is a shift that comes along with daily reflection on connection. Over time, this reflection can lend itself to a sense of belonging and, ultimately, to a sense of meaning and purpose as one understands one's own value as part of the fabric of others' lives.

Moments of high-quality social connections that provide meaning and purpose can be cultivated intentionally. In a client-centered coaching relationship, both client and coach reap the benefits that accrue from experiencing their close connection and sense of belonging.

Questions a Coach Would Ask

Open-ended inquiry, together with non-judgmental listening, provides Functional Medicine health coaches the opportunity to hear what clients need. Further, open-ended inquiry regarding their personal narratives provides clients with the opportunity to rewrite their story, incorporating strengths and redemptive features. Here are open-ended questions Functional Medicine health coaches may find valuable in supporting clients:

- When did you last feel well?
  This extremely important question in Functional Medicine takes the client back to a time before things changed from good to bad. The answer may elicit clues regarding triggering events that contributed to the onset of symptoms.
- What happened then?
- Was there anything going on in your life at that time that might have precipitated this illness, pain, or symptom?

These questions give clients permission to recall that connection and allow the client to connect symptoms with stressors or life changes.

- What impact have your symptoms had on your life?
  Asking such a powerful question can awaken within the client a desire to change course and use his or her strengths to create a better future.
- What do you want to do?
- What are you ready to do?
- What is the best way for me to coach you?
- Would you like to hear a suggestion?

Advocating and inspiring, Functional Medicine health coaches make specific suggestions or direct clients to resources that may help them. However, in contrast to the expert, the coach always asks the client for permission and respects his or her wishes.

By asking clients if they'd like a suggestion, the coach allows the client to either accept or reject the invitation. Contrast that with the professional, who acts as an expert and tells the individual directly what to do.

Notice how you felt while reading the questions listed above. How did your reaction compare with the emotions you experience when someone is ordering you to do something? This is the difference a client-centered approach can make.

Take the Connection: Functional Medicine and Client-Centered Coaching

Sally Morsbach, Pennsylvania, USA

I strongly believe in taking ownership. People often say, "I know what would help me; I just don't know why I don't do it." We don't always have to understand why we "don't do it." I ask clients, "What would you want to put in place if you could just dream big? If there were no obstacles and nobody gave you a hard time, what would that look like?"

I love the invitation that people often have to make choices. I sense that people feel stuck in some way, so they're seeking someone to take them across the field. When they pass the ball to me, I pass it back to them, and we do it together.

I say to my clients, "How are you taking care of yourself? Are you eating well? Are you sleeping well? Tell me more about your habits." Then I invite them to reflect on how they are doing with all that stuff. I'm not a fan of offering suggestions or encouraging people to do things that I haven't already tried.

I usually tell my clients when I meet them, "I have a lot of stories I could tell you, but I know nothing about yours. So I'm inviting you to teach me about you, and in that process, we'll journey together." When someone is struggling with an issue, I say, "Would you like me to share a story of someone else who dealt with something similar?" I invite their answer.

I work very collaboratively and I share. I'm pretty self-revealing, because if someone asks me a question, I want to model honesty and transparency.

Kara Badgley, Ohio, USA

I ask clients what they are doing currently for their care plan that they really believe in, that feels good to them, that they are interested in, and that is currently reasonable for them. These questions help clients identify where they are now and where they want to go next.

Leading by example was the biggest lesson the family I was coaching learned. No more separate meals. No more having the child eat alone. The parents joined in and did what was required to heal the child. Through leading by example, they were able to lead their son out of extreme picky eating. As an added benefit, the parents lost weight and no longer needed acid reflux medication. Within a year, their son had no behavioral goals on his individualized educational plan at school — only learning goals. Before, he had ONLY had behavioral goals.

When I first started working with families with autism, I was hell-bent on them understanding what I thought was best: NO gluten, NO casein, etc. I quickly learned I was turning people away from me. They couldn't hear what I had to offer because they weren't ready for this step. I've learned it's important that the family feels supported with what they are currently doing and chooses the next step from this place of feeling supported and cared for.

To gather myself before time with a client, I close my eyes. I breathe. I ask that I say the right thing at the right time for the client to hear, to discover exactly what they need at this exact moment.

Anne Caterino, Pennsylvania, USA

I was assigned a particular client through the Functional Medicine Coaching Center — a middle-aged male who had certainly had his share of health issues over the course of his life. Through working with a Functional Medicine doctor, he found out about our coaching center. He really struggled with sugar cravings, which caused him to awaken in the middle of the night. That's what he struggled with the most, so that's what he wanted help with. He also seemed to have a limited social support network and a lot of work-related stress.

We started working on his diet and the hypoglycemia, and he was really motivated. However, he would try to tackle a lot at once. He wanted to exercise but struggled with fatigue. Initially, I tried to ensure that he wasn't overwhelming himself with too many goals because he was so motivated. But then I decided to honor his motivation and rolled with it. About halfway through our sessions, he realized that when he exercised, he had more energy. He was able to breathe deeply and fully and concentrated on his breath when he was exercising. This awareness led to a discussion about deep breathing and oxygenation. He began doing more deep breathing techniques throughout the day, which opened up a whole new world for him in terms of not just relaxation, but decreasing fatigue and increasing energy.

I think he truly felt that he had a partner in health. He told me that before his visits with his Functional Medicine doctor, no one had ever looked at his illnesses from a root-cause approach. I became his ally in delving underneath the symptoms and using the positive psychology and the mind-body work to take it to the next level.

Shelby Garay, California, USA
I just love the energy that comes with coaching — I love that connection. People realize, "Wow, nobody's going to pressure me or tell me what to do." This allows them to take baby steps toward progress. For example, one client shared with me that he didn't think he was doing as much as he should and wasn't being the best client. Using strengths-spotting, I pointed out to him all the things he *did* do that really did add up, and he was amazed. I love helping people see that they can do this with little steps at a time and that it's going to help them.

Lawrence Robbins, Hong Kong, China
I give the client lots of time to chat, to listen, and to just feel like they have someone who's there — who actually hears them. They don't necessarily experience that when they meet one-on-one with their practitioner because the appointment times are so short. They're rushed in and rushed out, and they often leave feeling like they really weren't heard, so to speak.

Nowadays, patients have so much that's accessible to them via the Internet. I don't know many patients anymore who come to a doctor's appointment, listen to everything the doctor has to say, and walk out saying, "Well, I'm going to do everything the doctor says because the doctor is the expert and knows best what I should do." Instead, they listen to the provider, go home, and do their own research through Google.

I talk to patients quite often about this, and I encourage them to research, but I warn them to be mindful of their sources. I urge them to make sure that whatever they're reading — whatever they're investigating — comes from a reputable source, and I give them some examples of what they might find in Dr. Google versus a reputable source.

Veronica Lim, London, United Kingdom

My client was a middle-aged woman who was overweight and suffering from allergies. Over the years, she'd been on increasingly more potent allergy medications. She was feeling lethargic and really didn't know what to do. When she decided to work with me, she said she just felt a complete inability to eat and exercise the way she wanted to. With a history of yo-yo dieting, she didn't know what to do anymore. Her children were young, and she wanted more energy to keep up with them.

When we started working together, she identified her goals, one of which was to lose 24 pounds. In the end, however, she decided to reorient her goals, as what she really wanted was to feel alive and vital. She began focusing on eating nutritious food rather than counting calories and found that she had energy. However, she found it hard to let go of the diet mentality and returned to eating as little as possible rather than eating what was nutritious. The turning point came when I asked, "How did you feel when you were focused on eating healthy foods rather than eating to lose weight?" Within 24 hours, she was back on track, full of energy. I think that really helped her shift, as she realized that the adage "a calorie is just a calorie" is not correct.

It was a bit of a challenge to stay with the coach approach because she was very much in the place in which she just wanted someone to tell her what to do. To use the client-centered process with her, I asked, "In the last two weeks, how has your energy been? What were you doing differently in those two weeks, what have you been doing differently in the last few days, and what do you think the connection is?" With new awareness, she said, "The difference is that I went back to skimping on my eating."

Because of her allergies, I asked her about an elimination diet quite early in our conversation. This was simply to test the water — to see how ready she was to make some big changes in the way she was eating. She really didn't want to know at the time, but after making the connection between healthy eating and energy, she asked, "How can I find out more about the elimination diet?" I pointed her toward a resource, and the next time we spoke, she had already started it.

She literally took the bull by the horns and told me, "Okay, I'm just running with this, and I'm just going to do this, and I know that the first few weeks are going to be tough, but I'm really going to do this." She then brought her husband on board. I gave her some of the IFM resources, including the Cardiometabolic Food Plan and recipe book, and said, "Here's a resource you can study to see what healthy eating looks like." She and her husband loved some of the recipes.

I think one of the key questions I asked her was "What is going to make the biggest difference for you to keep with this new way of eating?" As a result of that question, she discovered that her main tool would be making sure that she was organized and that she planned ahead of time. She said, "If I don't keep myself organized and if I don't plan ahead of time, it just goes out the window." Another takeaway was preparing for the inevitable setback by saying, "It's okay. When I fall off, I can just get back on again."

———

For practitioners who enroll in the Functional Medicine Coaching Academy from traditional clinical backgrounds, the client-centered model of treatment may seem counterintuitive. They often can't resist the temptation to offer advice or recommend a remedy. But this is exactly the point: Treatment alone doesn't *heal* people. Coaches do not motivate people. Individuals find motivation from within and embark on their own unique healing journey. The coach goes along for the ride.

Coaching has been likened to dancing with a partner. We encourage Functional Medicine health coaches to trust their instincts and ability to connect with clients — to improvise, find a state of flow in which they lose all sense of time and place, and dance in the moment. This dance with clients contains no predetermined choreography. The coach lets the client lead but sometimes takes the lead by providing feedback, sharing observations, or offering suggestions if the client grants permission. By dancing in the moment, both the coach and the client experience a high-quality connection — an alliance that fosters belonging.

Chapter 8: Step into Meaning and Purpose

"Everyone has his own specific vocation or mission in life; everyone must carry out a concrete assignment that demands fulfillment. Therein he cannot be replaced, nor can his life be repeated, thus, everyone's task is as unique as his specific opportunity to implement it." — Viktor E. Frankl, author

Why Purpose Matters

While diet and lifestyle choices directly impact one's physical health, we strongly believe that the key ingredient that contributes to both physical and mental well-being consists of finding meaning and purpose. We've seen the transformational power of finding meaning and purpose both in ourselves and in others, including FMCA students (whose stories we'll share at the end of this chapter) and their clients.

In Man's Search for Meaning, Viktor Frankl writes about the possibility of finding meaning despite suffering. A Viennese psychiatrist, Frankl was imprisoned for three years in Auschwitz, a Nazi concentration camp. The prisoners in the camps lost everything, but some continued to believe that their lives had meaning and showed resilience to suffering. Those prisoners who found meaning believed that something in the future was expected of them, such as telling the world about the horrors of the concentration camp. Frankl observed that those who knew the "why" for their existence could withstand almost anything. He concluded that individuals have a will for meaning and that this drive to find meaning in life is our primary motivational force.

Dr. Barbara Fredrickson provided scientific validation for Dr. Frankl's conclusions through her research on hedonic well-being versus eudaimonic well-being. Hedonic well-being centers around positive emotional experiences, while eudaimonic well-being refers to finding meaning in life, believing one has a contribution to make to society, and experiencing life as full of opportunities for growth and transformation. Both states are important, as people who experience more positive emotions experience more meaning and those who experience more meaning experience more positive emotions.

Fredrickson found that eudaimonic well-being more directly connects to a healthy pattern of gene expression than hedonic well-being. These results were replicated across two different samples using different measures. Her later research showed that positive emotions are also associated with healthy gene expression, but only to the extent that they affect eudaimonic well-being. Fredrickson believes that eudaimonic well-being is the active ingredient that is most directly related to good health.

Given the importance of eudaimonic well-being for physical health, one of the most important roles of a Functional Medicine health coach is helping clients find meaning and purpose. While goal-setting and behavior change are also central to the coaching process, how can coaches help clients sustain the changes they make? For goals and intentional change to be sustained, they must be rooted in meaning and purpose. That process involves the use of positive emotional attractors (PEAs).

Use Positive Emotional Attractors

The concept of a positive emotional attractor was developed by Richard Boyatzis of Case Western Reserve University and derives from the Intentional Change Theory. The PEA relates to the personal hopes, possibilities, strengths, and optimism that we all have, while a negative emotional attractor (NEA) relates to fears, shortcomings, and pessimism.

According to the Intentional Change Theory, goal setting works best when supported by mindful reflection on what matters most to the individual. The Functional Medicine health coach asks questions such as "What matters most?" and "What is your personal vision?" Intentional change begins when the ideal self is connected to the change process. The change process, therefore, becomes associated with one's personal passions and a belief in future possibilities.

The physiological effects of the PEA and the NEA are very different. In a research study by Dr. Anita Howard, coaches used the participant's own hopes, strengths, and desired future (PEAs) as an anchoring framework for a coaching session. These sessions began with a discussion of the client's personal vision followed by the coach's provision of support. In the NEA condition, coaches used the participant's current life circumstances and need for improvement as the anchoring framework. Howard found that participants in the PEA condition demonstrated significantly lower levels of negative emotion and focused more on personal interests and passions compared to those in the NEA condition.

When focusing on personal vision, we arouse parts of the brain associated with imagining and being open to new ideas, people, and emotions. Activating these neural circuits associated with openness and scanning the environment for possibilities activates the parasympathetic branch of the autonomic nervous system (PNS). Turning on the PNS means that we're in a state conducive to relaxation, renewal, and restoration, a state that fosters clear thinking and creativity. Focusing on one's ideal future, dreams, and personal vision allows for renewal of the body and mind. This process reverses the damaging effects of chronic stress and positively affects sustainability of the change effort.

In a 2010 study, Boyatzis and colleagues used functional magnetic resonance imaging (MRI) to study approaches to coaching. When university students were asked to dream about the future, the MRI showed that neural regions associated with imagining were activated. This activation was significantly greater than when the same subjects experienced a comparable coaching session that was focused on things they should have been doing, thereby arousing the negative emotional attractor. The PEA coaching session in this study involved one question: "What would your life be like ten years in the future if everything were ideal?" The NEA coaching involved questions about the students' current academic experience, such as "How are you doing in your courses? Are you doing all the readings and homework?"

Frequently bringing clients into awareness about their PEA can renew their openness to the possibilities of change, including new ideas and new emotions. Commitment to one's own positive identity and curiosity about one's potential for change drive the decision to change and the ability to stick with the change plan no matter what. Coaches help their clients unleash the power of their intrinsic motivation to change by helping them identify their PEA.

By accessing our PEAs, we gain insight into our meaning and purpose. In an interview recorded for FMCA students, Dr. Howard spoke about her personal interactions in the 1960s with many of the civil rights leaders. She witnessed how these individuals held onto their hopes and dreams to overcome the significant challenges they faced. Martin Luther King Jr.'s famous "I Have a Dream" speech, in which he so eloquently described his vision for the future, epitomizes how a PEA connects to meaning and purpose in life.

According to both Howard and Boyatzis, your vision, elicited when you access your PEA, moves you to sustain a desired change. The ideal self or personal vision becomes a driver of change by focusing the client's attention and energizing the client both psychologically and physiologically.

PEA can be aroused through compassion and gratitude and through a focus on values, virtues, oneness, mindfulness, and even playfulness. Beginning the coaching process and even each coaching session with a discussion of the client's core vision equips individuals to be more open and resilient during a discussion of needs for improvement.

Individuals are more motivated when they set vision-centered goals, even in the face of very difficult challenges. Boyatzis and Howard believe that for goal-setting to be motivational, it must help a person move into the joy and excitement of the positive emotional attractor. Arousing a sense of guilt and obligation does not lead to sustained change. Only through accessing the PEA and connecting to meaning and greater purpose can lasting change occur.

Questions a Coach Would Ask

Through open-ended questioning, clients may increase awareness of what brings them meaning and purpose and what type of future they desire. As a result, they may become motivated to make behavior changes. To elicit this awareness, the following questions may be helpful:

- What gives you meaning and purpose and makes life worthwhile?
- What brings you joy and contentment?
- What would your life be like if you were free of pain?
- Where would you like to be in five or ten years? What will you be doing that is different? How will you be feeling that is different from the way you're feeling now?
- How do you think I can help you, and what kinds of resources do you need?

By using questions like these to focus on both the eudaimonic factors and positive emotional attractors, coaches set the stage for the neural patterning of healing to take place in ways that may have been previously unavailable to clients.

When combined with a Functional Medicine approach, the transformative power of coaching that addresses meaning and purpose can halt the progression of chronic illnesses and, in many cases, reverse illness altogether.

Make the Connection: Step into Meaning and Purpose as a Functional Medicine Health Coach

Jennah Nelson, Ohio, USA

I have begun to live by the phrase "When you know better, you do better." Here I am on a mission to do better!

Looking back, I guess I could say functional nutrition has been an integral part of my life even before I knew what to call it. At 15, I was diagnosed as prediabetic. By working closely with my physician and reading nearly every piece of literature he handed me, I've been able to successfully stay diabetes-free for the last 15 years. Through nutrition, exercise, and a constant desire to learn, I warded off what is one of the greatest epidemics of my time and avoided becoming another statistic.

Flash forward to age 28, when I suffered a miscarriage. Devastated, I made it my mission to learn all that I could. After lots of blood work and more diagnostic discoveries, I learned that I was doing many things incorrectly, but I also realized they could all be corrected through nutrition and proper supplementation.

Shocked at some of the things I was discovering, I wondered how many other women were walking around making all the same mistakes I was and struggling through fertility treatments, not realizing the answer could be so much simpler. I started reading more and more, learning from my physician, and realizing how much my gut health and stress levels at work were ruining me. I knew I had to re-evaluate the way I was going through life and start taking my own health into my control. After finding out how imbalanced my gut microbiome was from years of taking proton pump inhibitors (for the acid reflux I developed from stress), I knew it was time to make a life change, so I did.

I spent the next six to seven months recovering from the emotional stresses of a miscarriage by becoming addicted to yoga. I changed everything I was taking, doing, and eating, as well as how I was living. What a sense of freedom I gained! I successfully became pregnant and now have a beautiful baby girl!

Shortly after giving birth to her and sharing my story with others, my vision became clear. I was sitting in my cubicle trudging through another unfulfilling work day, researching nutrition on the web, when I stumbled across a tweet from Dr. Mark Hyman (someone I've followed since I was 15). He was tweeting about FMCA. I emailed my physician asking what he thought, and he replied with one word: YES.

The next day I quit my job and made it my mission to throw everything I have into this career and help others. I get chills thinking about how awesome this is going to be, and I have so many ideas that I can't get them on paper fast enough.

Eileen Immerman, Wisconsin, USA
I'm probably one of the older coaching students, and I hear people say, "Why don't you just retire?" I tell them that this is going to be the most important thing I do, even if I do it for five years or for ten.

On my website, I have a post on inflammation. I inserted pictures from when I was first married, when my children were young, just before I got sick, and now that I'm well. This is my story. If even one person sees these and thinks, "You know what, I can do this too," then I've fulfilled my mission.

Nikki Dickerson, Texas, USA
I intend to make a career shift from high school assistant principal to health coach so that I can walk the path with others to their wellness. I am grateful for the fact that cancer entered my life to serve as the great "awakening" to changes that needed to be made in my life. However, I certainly intend to create an internal environment that the cancer will not want to return to.

Heather Aardema, Colorado, USA
This is my passion — I just have so much energy. It's a little bit odd for someone with two autoimmune diseases, but I really do have tremendous energy. Working in corporate America just didn't speak to my heart, but this program does, as does helping others. I look at the emotional well-being of my clients as most important. On a ten-point scale, where ten is

great and one is horrible, they started around three or four, and now they're between eight and ten.

You feel good when you've been the accountability partner, the ally, the idea generator, and the brainstormer. I believe part of why they're thriving is their relationship with me, and that gives me goose bumps.

In my corporate life, there was a separation between what I did on the job and my home life, and I don't want that separation. What's awesome about Functional Medicine health coaching is that there doesn't have to be a separation. What I'm learning about and applying to coaching I'm also using in my personal life. I just feel so fortunate to be in this program and to be where I am right now — In this day, in this time.

———

What most inspires us about our work at the Functional Medicine Coaching Academy is knowing that when we help coaches find well-being and connect them with a sense of purpose, they pay it forward by replicating this process with clients.

For the first time in recorded American history, the current generation's health prospects do not exceed that of their predecessors. However, we remain optimistic given the surging demand for Functional Medicine and the growth of patient-empowered healthcare. Increased commitment to action will come as more people experience a sense of purpose in their lives, which will enable them to make the decision to take back their health. We teach Functional Medicine health coaches to adopt these principles in their training. They find meaning and purpose when they join the growing Functional Medicine community and make a commitment to serve others.

Conclusion

Psychiatrist Alfred Adler believed that mental health is directly connected to the notion that every individual is an integral part of a larger social whole. True happiness, as well as meaning and purpose in life, derives from the experience of giving to a community.

According to Emily Esfahani Smith, a sense of belonging may be the most important driver of meaning. Belonging is simply the idea that you fit in a particular place; that you are needed there at this time. Belonging implies that your very presence is valuable, even if you "do" nothing.

A strong sense of belonging nurtures one's sense of purpose. When we acknowledge that we are valuable, we are believing we have a reason for existing — a purpose in our relationships.

While witnessing the horrors of Auschwitz, Victor Frankl realized that love and connection to others is the basis for a meaningful life. "Being human always points, and is directed to, something or someone other than oneself, be it a meaning to fulfill or another human being to encounter. The more one forgets himself by giving himself to a cause to serve or another person to love, the more human he is."

The visionary scientists and physicians who gave birth to and grew the Functional Medicine movement, including Dr. Jeffrey Bland and Dr. Mark Hyman, speak lovingly about the Functional Medicine community, using words such as "family" and "tribe" to describe the deep bonds that develop among those who share common values and aspirations. The

Institute for Functional Medicine faculty, many of whom also serve on our FMCA faculty, and the growing number of Functional Medicine practitioners, also attest to the power of this community.

Discovering the Functional Medicine approach to understanding and treating chronic disease was a life-altering experience for us, our students, and our students' clients. But the experience of joining the Functional Medicine community and making meaningful connections with like-minded individuals proved to be even more powerful. It was transformative, giving so many of us a renewed sense of meaning and purpose.

Meaningful relationships, connection to others, and a sense of belonging appear again and again in the stories we collected. In addition to ties to family and friends, those we interviewed felt deeply connected to their clients and the Functional Medicine community. Out of their love for Functional Medicine, they found meaning and purpose — a desire to serve others and spread the word about the Functional Medicine approach to healthcare.

Compassion lies at the heart of belonging. When we open our hearts to others and approach them with love and kindness, we enrich both those around us and ourselves. If we want to find meaning in our lives, the fastest way to begin is by reaching out to others and reminding ourselves that we belong here.

Without exception, those who want to become Functional Medicine health coaches and apply for admission to FMCA have a passion for helping others and a desire to serve that comes from a deep sense of compassion.

If, after reading this book, you're considering a career as a Functional Medicine health coach, you'll need three important prerequisites: mindfulness, hope, and compassion. Richard Boyatzis describes these three elements as the key to positive interactions. By bringing mindfulness, hope, and compassion to every coaching encounter, you will help change lives for the better.

We hope that you will join the growing Functional Medicine community, whether as a Functional Medicine health coach, a client, or both. Belonging to our family can bring you meaning and purpose, better health and well-being, and the knowledge, tools, and skills to create health around the globe.

No one can convey the power of the Functional Medicine community and becoming a Functional Medicine health coach better than our students:

Anindita Rungta, Mumbai, India
Clients want to have someone who will lead them along the way and just listen. They just want to speak to someone who understands, who's there with them, and, of course, who can guide them.

The fact that I can bring all this to someone else who is going through what I have been through gives me immense pleasure and deep purpose that I look forward to for the rest of my life.

Functional Medicine health coaching is like the first drop in the ocean right now in India. I have not marketed myself, but just by speaking to a few people, I already have quite a few clients. This tells me that there is so much demand everywhere for this.

Heather Shover, Texas, USA

What kept me going when I was sick was getting the word out to people that there's a different way to heal. That's my passion — my life purpose.

I meet regularly with a group here in Dallas. It's a growing group, and I love that. I talk about it a lot, and people who attend often bring back a friend or two the next month who may also have a chronic disease. Everyone gets to know each other and shares their individual journeys, and bonding takes place. I have the opportunity to explain that there is a better way to do this that will get an individual healthy faster.

I think there's so much healing in community.

Jesse Proctor, North Carolina, USA

Functional Medicine has really lifted me up and out of the fog and gloom of my illness. Since I've been sick, I have a lot of friends and acquaintances in my community that I connect with about their own physical struggles. It just so happened that this incredible, thoughtful, introspective community has popped up around disease. Something very wonderful and transformative has come from a lot of people experiencing chronic issues with their bodies or minds. I find myself in the position of offering information and a listening ear to a lot of people who are feeling sick. Their story is my story. I feel it so much and want to be able to provide them with more information and help them achieve their goals. I wanted more knowledge on how to do that, and FMCA was the perfect next step.

I get a real sense of belonging from being able to connect with people, especially about their health issues, because these issues dramatically affect people's experience of being alive and what that looks like to them. When I get to share my experience with other people struggling with physical and mental ailments, share information with them, and help them find the wisdom within to improve their circumstances, I feel deeply fulfilled and deeply connected to the world and the life inside me. Just because that's where I can see it, through my own experience, that's where I am finding purpose.

Heather Aardema, Colorado, USA
It's been really fun for me since I left corporate America. I created a health and well-being meetup group called Well Being Alive that meets once a month in Denver. I find speakers and people come, supporting and inspiring each other. It's not a pity party. Everyone that comes wants to feel better. We go around the table talking about our favorite brands, books, blogs, and so forth.

Everyone takes notes furiously, and it really is all about inspiration. A lot of the women have autoimmune diseases or have had cancer. Their spouses think, "Oh, my wife is on this crazy diet. What the heck is this?" No one wants to talk about it. I created a safe space in which everyone can open up their hearts and be themselves and not be judged. It's just like a group hug!

Liz Novy, Ohio, USA

My client's physician made health coaching part of my client's comprehensive program. He was very interested in the process, and, with her consent, he shared with me his plan of care, really getting me involved in his goals for her. The fact that I was part of a collaborative care team really made a difference for her.

The important part of coaching is not the content but the process of creating that positive connection with others. That can be healing and motivating, and it's a great side benefit of work if that's part of what contributes to the coach's own health and well-being.

Raewyn Guerrero, London, United Kingdom

Coaching is a circle of support. We're working together to give the client the best experience possible.

I do believe that everyone should have a coach. Friends or social networks are great, but it's nice to have someone dedicated specifically to you. You can work stuff out and bounce stuff off them. I can see no downsides.

I feel blessed and even grateful that all my own health issues have led me here — to the crest of a wave that's going to change the world, one person at a time.

Shelby Garay, California, USA

It would have been nice to have had a cheerleader — someone to say, "You know what? Your instincts are right. You're doing great."

It's exciting to be on the cusp of this whole new evolution of medicine, and I see endless possibilities. When I share just a little bit about Functional Medicine with people I meet, they ask me how they can learn more. I just really want to help people discover their own motivation to achieve their best health.

True happiness comes from helping other people, engaging with them, and just making their lives a little brighter with every interaction.

Raluca Stanescu, London, United Kingdom

I believed in Functional Medicine with all my heart and became unstoppable in my fight to get my health back. After managing to reverse rheumatoid arthritis, I decided to change my life completely and help other people regain their health through Functional Medicine. I left the corporate environment and started my own business of Functional Medicine health coaching and motivational speaking.

Becoming a Functional Medicine health coach is a dream come true. I have always been passionate about people, food, and health and am incredibly grateful to be able to follow my passion and transform it into my day job. When you do what you truly love, you get an immense energy, which makes you feel unstoppable. Being able to help other people is the best feeling anyone could ever have.

We only learn to appreciate the true value of health when we are close to losing it, but the body has immense recovery capabilities if we are strong enough to make the right lifestyle choices. This is the reason I love Functional Medicine health coaching. It is the right link between people and healthy lifestyle choices.

My dream is becoming a worldwide ambassador for Functional Medicine, motivating and empowering people to overcome their physical and emotional challenges while helping them fight chronic illnesses and get their health back.

Functional Medicine health coaching is the future of healthcare and well-being as people need more and more support to change their behavior and make healthier lifestyle choices. This is only the beginning of an impressive journey.

Elizabeth Grimm, Nevada, USA

After going through years and years of treatment, I can relate to others who feel ostracized by the medical community. I want to let them know health is possible. I am excited to walk this healing journey with others.

Veronica Lim, London, United Kingdom

After I discovered Functional Medicine, I realized that it's an addictive path.

Daniela Cook, Dubai, United Arab Emirates

I'm very happy with my FMCA community and being with like-minded people. I don't have to see them every day, but just knowing they're out there is quite good for me.

I'd like to believe that we can slowly change the world, one country at a time.

Morgan Mitchell, Maine, USA

My name is not rheumatoid arthritis; my name is Morgan Mitchell. That's what I felt like saying to the doctor who diagnosed me in Romania in 2013 at the age of 22. "This is a chronic disease that you will have for the rest of your life," she said as she slid a Methotrexate prescription across the table.

Fast forward a year and a half when I returned to that clinic to be reunited with the doctor. She looked pleased to see that my inflammation was gone and applauded me for taking the medication she had prescribed. Her pleased expression slipped into puzzlement when I explained that I felt better than ever and that I had not taken any medication. I explained that food and lifestyle had been my medication. She replied that what I was doing was dangerous and that I should reconsider taking the medication. I wished her well and went on my way.

This is my story — a story I share with countless people around the world. When I was sick, frustrated, and bewildered, I craved the support of someone who could guide and encourage me along my long and winding road to wellness. Long nights of research and Google searches brought me to the realization that if I really wanted to get well, my path to recovery was not within the walls of the traditional medical system. From that moment on, I made a silent vow to find a way to be a part of the solution. Becoming a Functional Medicine Certified Health Coach could not be more in alignment with this intention.

Appendix: Resources

Book a FREE Functional Medicine Health Coaching Session

This book comes with one FREE Functional Medicine health coaching session.
To set up your free session, text COACHING to 847-220-6353 or email intakecoordinator@functionalmedicinecoaching.org, and instructions will be sent to you.

Get a Functional Medicine Health Coach

Would you like to work with one of our apprentice coaches through the Functional Medicine Coaching Center? Take advantage of a first session at no charge. Additional sessions are extremely affordable. Preliminary results from outcome data show that clients who work with our apprentice coaches achieve positive results in a short period of time.

To register, go to: http://www.coachingcenter.functionalmedicinecoaching.org/.

Become a Functional Medicine Health Coach

Are you passionate about helping others? Do you have a calling to serve? Are you ready for a career change? Would you like to add Functional Medicine health coaching to your existing healthcare or wellness practice? Do you want to learn the principles of Functional Medicine and positive psychology to improve your own health or the health of your family? After reading the stories in this book, are you considering becoming a Functional Medicine Certified Health Coach? We invite you to join our growing community.

To apply, visit https://www.functionalmedicinecoaching.org/.

Find a Functional Medicine Practitioner

Are you interested in working with a Functional Medicine practitioner (physician, chiropractor, etc.) that has been trained through The Institute for Functional Medicine? To find a practitioner in your area, visit https://www.functionalmedicine.org/.

Additional Websites

Functional Forum, presented by Evolution of Medicine, is the world's largest Functional Medicine gathering. On the first Monday of each month, practitioners and coaches gather in meet-up groups around the world to network and hear about the latest Functional Medicine research and practice development strategies. To learn more, visit http://functionalforum.com/

The VIA Institute on Character offers a free strengths survey. This survey, taken by more than four million people worldwide, reveals the strengths one can leverage to create health goals. To learn more, visit http://www.viacharacter.org/

The International Consortium for Health & Wellness Coaching (ICHWC), formerly known as the National Consortium for Credentialing Health and Wellness Coaches (NCCHWC) http://ichwc.org/

The International Coach Federation (ICF) http://www.coachfederation.org/

Handouts

Functional Medicine Matrix

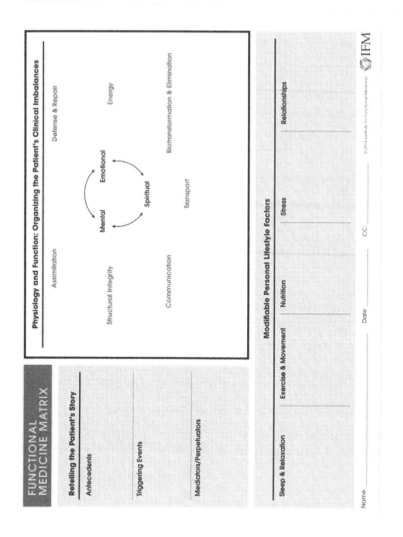

Go to http://bit.ly/2nqN4YL

Phytonutrient Spectrum

Phytonutrient Spectrum Foods

RED

Foods				Benefits	
Apples	Cranberries	Pomegranate	Rhubarb	Anti-cancer	Gastrointestinal health
Beans (adzuki,	Cherries	Potatoes	Rooibos tea	Anti-inflammatory	Heart health
kidney, red)	Grapefruit (pink)	Radicchio	Tomato	Cell protection	Hormone health
Beets	Goji berries	Radishes	Watermelon		Liver health
Bell peppers	Grapes	Raspberries			
Blood oranges	Onions	Strawberries			
	Plums	Sweet red peppers			

ORANGE

Foods				Benefits	
Apricots	Mango	Pumpkin	Tangerines	Anti-cancer	Reduced mortality
Bell peppers	Nectarine	Squash (acorn,	Turmeric root	Anti-bacterial	Reproductive health
Cantaloupe	Orange	butternut, summer,	Yams	Immune health	Skin health
Carrots	Papaya	winter)		Cell protection	Source of vitamin A
	Persimmons	Sweet potato			

YELLOW

Foods				Benefits	
Apple	Bell peppers	Lemon	Starfruit	Anti-cancer	Eye health
Asian pears	Corn	Millet	Succotash	Anti-inflammatory	Heart health
Banana	Corn-on-the-cob	Pineapple	Summer squash	Cell protection	Skin health
	Ginger root			Cognition	Vascular health

GREEN

Foods				Benefits	
Apples	Bok choy	Green peas	Okra	Anti-inflammatory	Skin health
Artichoke	Broccoli	Green tea	Olives	Brain health	Hormone balance
Asparagus	Broccolini	Greens (arugula, beet,	Pears	Cell protection	Heart health
Avocado	Brussels sprouts	chard, sweet chard	Snow peas		Liver health
Bamboo sprouts	Cabbage	collard, dandelion,	Watercress		
Bean sprouts	Celery	kale, lettuce, mustard,	Zucchini		
Bell peppers	Cucumbers	spinach, turnip)	Anti-cancer		
Bitter melon	Edamame/soy beans	Limes			
	Green beans				

BLUE/PURPLE/BLACK

Foods				Benefits	
Bell peppers	Cabbage	Grapes	Prunes	Anti-cancer	Cognitive health
Berries (bilberries, black,	Carrots	Kale	Raisins	Anti-inflammatory	Heart health
boysenberries,	Cauliflower	Olives	Rice (black	Cell protection	Liver health
huckleberries,	Eggplant	Plums	or purple)		
marionberries)	Figs	Potatoes			

WHITE/TAN/BROWN

Foods				Benefits	
Apples	Dates	Mushrooms	Shallots	Anti-cancer	Heart health
Applesauce	Garlic	Nuts (almonds, cashews,	Soy	Anti-microbial	Hormone health
Bean dips	Ginger	pecans, walnuts)	Tahini	Cell protection	Liver health
Cauliflower	Jicama	Onions	Tea (black, white)	Gastrointestinal	
Cocoa	Legumes (chickpeas,	Pears	Whole grains	health	
Coconut	dried beans or peas,	Sauerkraut	(barley, brown, oat,		
Coffee	hummus, lentils,	Seeds (flax, hemp,	oat, quinoa, rye,		
	peanuts, refried beans,	pumpkin, sesame,	spelt, wheat)		
	low-fat)	sunflower)			

© 2014 The Institute for Functional Medicine

Go to http://bit.ly/2o9VGzO

Functional Medicine Timeline

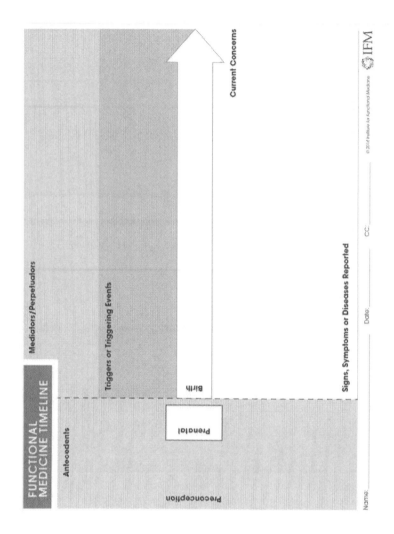

Go to http://bit.ly/2nO68LL

Acknowledgements

We could not have created this book without the many wonderful people in our lives: family, friends, colleagues, students, and clients.

To our loving spouses, Alan Scheinbaum and Rob Klein: We extend our heartfelt thanks for all the things you do, both large and small, and for your patience in bearing with us as we took so much time away from being with you to develop the book. To our children, Laura and Keith Harrison and Carly Scheinbaum, as well as fiancé Alex Valvassori and baby girl Klein (who will be born after we go to print): You give us meaning and purpose and are the light of our lives.

How can we ever fully thank our collaboration partner, the Institute for Functional Medicine? Laurie Hofmann, Dr. Kristi Hughes, Dr. Patrick Hanaway, Dr. Robert Luby, Dr. Dan Lukaczer, Andie Crosby, Sally Priest, and many others believe in FMCA and our mission and lend support in so many ways.

We give thanks to the dedicated experts who comprise our board of advisors: Dr. Mark Hyman, Laurie Hofmann, Dr. David Jones, Dr. Kristi Hughes, Dr. Beth Frates, Monique Class, Lyra Heller, Jennifer Newton, and Dr. Lynn Johnson. Your support, guidance, and encouragement are much appreciated.

Without the world-renowned experts who comprise our faculty, we would not have earned recognition as an institution known for academic excellence. We are in awe of your brilliance.

A huge thank-you goes out to everyone on the FMCA team: Jennifer Champion, Liz Novy, Andrea Cook, Stefanie Greene, Olivia Pelaez, Carly Scheinbaum, Ginna Johnson, Roberta Holstein, Connie Swan, Elizabeth McHugh, Caryn Larrinaga, Anthony Stewart, Patty Campbell, Andrew Carter, and Kristy Johnson. We appreciate your many contributions, too numerable to mention.

We want to recognize our course facilitators: Holly Ladd, Gabrielle Grandell, Kara Badgley, Shelby Garay, Alexandra Marin, Jessica Talley-Haynes, Amber Letz, Gina Lockwood-Sheehan, Karen Roach, Kari Schadler, Cherri Schleicher, Gina Sundberg, Patty Bean, Mare Tomaski, Mahnaz Malik, Veronica Lim, and Lydia Flores. You work tirelessly to ensure that all students feel heard and connected, and we're so grateful that you are part of the team.

It takes a community to write a book. First and foremost, we want to thank Dr. Mark Hyman for writing the foreword. No matter what else is going on in your busy life, you always make time to support FMCA's mission. We're grateful for everything that you do to promote the growth of Functional Medicine and Functional Medicine health coaching. Our editor, Kristen Domingue, did a masterful job of taking our words and making them sing on the page, and Kelly Stock helped immensely to get the manuscript whipped into shape. We also want to thank Samantha Ferrara for designing the book cover, Barry Schimmel for providing proofreading and publishing support, and Mary Agnes Antonopoulos for working her magic to make sure the messages in this book are communicated to a larger audience.

Most importantly, we want to acknowledge the students of the Functional Medicine Coaching Academy. Without our students, there would be no school. These incredible individuals came to FMCA out of a desire to serve others and pursue their passion for changing people's lives through the power of Functional Medicine. They shared their personal stories to spread the message about how they healed themselves through Functional Medicine and how their lives were transformed through the decision to become a Functional Medicine Certified Health Coach. Each one of your stories moved us and spoke to us. All had value, and narrowing down which ones to include in this book was quite a difficult task.

A profound thank-you also goes to the clients who signed up to be coached by our apprentices through the Functional Medicine Coaching Center. We hope that you experienced the power of Functional Medicine health coaching and are grateful that you are now part of the Functional Medicine community.

With heartfelt gratitude,
Sandi and Elyse

Books

Coaching Basics

Arloski, M. (2009). Wellness Coaching for Lasting Lifestyle Change. Duluth, MN: Whole Person Associates, Inc.

Brann, A. (2015). Neuroscience for Coaches. London, United Kingdom: Kogan Page Limited.

Dass, R. & Gorman, P. (1985). How Can I Help?: Stories and Reflections on Service. New York, NY: Alfred A. Knopf.

Deci, E. & Flaste, R. (1996). Why We Do What We Do. London, England: Penguin Books.

Grant, A. M. & Stober, D. R. (2006). Evidence Based Coaching Handbook: Putting Best Practices to Work for Your Clients. Hoboken, NJ: John Wiley & Sons, Inc.

Jordan, M. & Livingstone, J. (2013). Coaching versus psychotherapy in health and wellness: Overlap, dissimilarities and the potential for collaboration. Global Advances in Health and Medicine, 2(4): 44-51.

Jordan, M. (2012). Fast track to health, well-being and happiness: The emerging profession of health coaches. Anthropology, March.

Jordan, M. (2013). Health coaching for the underserved. Global Advances in Health and Medicine, 2(3): 75-82.

Miller, W. (2012). Motivational Interviewing: Helping People Change (3rd ed.). New York, NY: The Guilford Press

Moore, M. (2012). Coaching Psychology Manual. Philadelphia, PA: Lippincott Williams & Wilkins.

Newberg, A. & Waldman, M. R. (2012). Words Can Change Your Brain. New York, NY: Penguin Group.

Prochaska, J (2006). Changing for Good. New York, NY: First Collins Paperback.

White, W. R. (2007). In Over Our Heads: Meditations on Grace. Augsburg Fortress.

Whitworth, L. (2007). Co-Active Coaching: New Skills for Coaching People Toward Success in Work and Life. Mountain View, CA: Davies-Black Pub.

Cookbooks

Edelson, M. & Katz, R. (2004). One Bite at a Time. Berkeley, CA: Ten Speed Press.

Edelson, M. & Katz, R. (2013). The Longevity Kitchen. Berkeley, CA: Ten Speed Press.

Edelson, M. & Katz, R. (2015). The Healthy Mind Cookbook. Berkeley, CA: Ten Speed Press.

Edelson, M., Katz, R. & Tomassi, M. (2009). The Cancer-Fighting Kitchen. Berkeley, CA: Ten Speed Press.

Hyman, M. (2015). The Blood Sugar Solution 10-Day Detox Diet Cookbook. New York, NY: Little, Brown and Company.

Katz, R. (2016). Clean Soups: Simple, Nourishing Recipes for Health and Vitality. Emeryville, CA: Ten Speed Press.

Malterre, T. & Segersten, A. (2014). The Whole Life Nutrition Cookbook. New York, NY: Grand Central Life & Style.

McGruther, J. (2014). The Nourishing Kitchen: Farm-to-Table Recipes for the Traditional Foods Lifestyle. Berkley, CA: Ten Speed Press.

Perlmutter, D. (2014). Grain Brain Cookbook: More Than 150 Life-Changing Gluten-Free Recipes to Transform Your Health. New York, NY: Little, Brown and Company.

Wagner, E. L. (2014). Smoothie Secrets Revealed: A Guide to Enhance Your Health. Lake Zurich, IL: My Kitchen Shrink Inc.

Wahls, T. (2017). The Wahl's Protocol Cooking for Life: The Revolutionary Modern Paleo Plan to Treat All Chronic Autoimmune Conditions. Garden City, New York: Avery Publishing.

Functional Medicine/Healthcare

Axe, J. (2016). Eat Dirt: Why Leaky Gut May Be the Root Cause of Your Health Problems and 5 Surprising Steps to Cure It. New York, NY: Harper Wave.

Bland, J. S. (2014). The Disease Delusion: Conquering the Causes of Chronic Illness for a Healthier, Longer, and Happier Life. New York, NY: HarperOne.

Blum, S. & Bender, M. (2013). The Immune System Recovery Plan: A Doctor's 4-Step Program to Treat Autoimmune Disease. New York, NY: Scribner.

Brogan, K. (2016). A Mind of Your Own. New York, NY: HarperCollins.

Fitzgerald, K. (2016). Methylation Diet and Lifestyle. [e-book].

Guarneri, M. (2006). The Heart Speaks. New York, NY: Touchstone.

Hyman, M. (2012). The Blood Sugar Solution 10-Day Detox Diet: Activate Your Body's Natural Ability to Burn Fat and Lose Weight Fast. New York, NY: Little, Brown and Company.

Hyman, M. (2016). Eat Fat, Get Thin. New York, NY: Little, Brown and Company.

Johnson, L. (2010). The Healing Power of Sleep. Head Acre Press.

Katz, D. L. (2013). Disease-Proof: The Remarkable Truth About What Makes Us Well. Garden City, New York: Avery Publishing.

Kharrazian, D. (2010). Why Do I Still Have Thyroid Symptoms? When My Lab Tests Are Normal: a Revolutionary Breakthrough in Understanding Hashimoto's Disease and Hypothyroidism. Carlsbad, CA: Elephant Press Books.

Maskell, J. (2016). The Evolution of Medicine: Join the Movement to Solve Chronic Disease and Fall Back in Love with Medicine. [ebook]. Retrieved from https://www.amazon.com/ Evolution-Medicine-Movement-Chronic-Disease-ebook.

Minich, D. (2016). Whole Detox. New York, NY: HarperCollins.

Mullin, G. E. & Swift, K. M. (2011). The Inside Tract: Your Good Gut Guide to Great Digestive Health. New York, NY: Rodale Books.

Myers, A. (2015). The Autoimmune Solution: Prevent and Reverse the Full Spectrum of Inflammatory Symptoms and Diseases. New York NY: HarperOne.

Myers, A. (2016). The Thyroid Connection: Why You Feel Tired, Brain-Fogged, and Overweight -- And How to Get Your Life Back. New York, NY: Little, Brown and Company.

O'Bryan, T. (2016). The Autoimmune Fix: How to Stop the Hidden Autoimmune Damage That Keeps You Sick, Fat, and Tired Before It Turns Into Disease. Seattle, WA: Amazon Digital Services LLC.

Osborne, P. (2016). No Grain, No Pain: A 30-Day Diet for Eliminating the Root Cause of Chronic Pain. New York, NY: Touchstone/Simon and Schuster.

Perlmutter, D. (2013). Grain Brain: The Surprising Truth About Wheat, Carbs, and Sugar. New York, NY: Little, Brown and Company.

Perlmutter, D. (2015). Brain Maker: The Power of Gut Microbes to Heal and Protect Your Brain – for Life. New York, NY: Little, Brown and Company.

Perlmutter, D. (2016). The Grain Brain Whole Life Plan: Boost Brain Performance, Lose Weight, and Achieve Optimal Health. New York, NY: Little, Brown and Company.

Quinn, S. (2010). Textbook of Functional Medicine. Institute for Functional Medicine.

Romm, A. (2017). The Adrenal Thyroid Revolution: A Proven 4-Week Program to Rescue Your Metabolism, Hormones, Mind & Mood. New York, NY: HarperCollins Publishers.

Scheinbaum, S. (2015). Stop Panic Attacks in 10 Easy Steps: Using Functional Medicine to Calm Your

Mind and Body with Drug-Free Techniques. London, UK: Jessica Kingsley Publishers.

Smith, J. M. (2012). Genetic Roulette: The Gamble of Our Lives. Jeffrey M. Smith: Author.

Sult, T. A. (2013). Just Be Well: A Book for Seekers of Vibrant Health. Highland Park, IL: Round Table Companies.

Topol, Eric. (2015). The Patient Will See You Now. New York, NY: Basic Books.

Wahls, T. (2014). The Wahl's Protocol: A Radical New Way to Treat All Chronic Autoimmune Conditions Using Paleo Principles and Functional Medicine. New York, NY: Avery.

Wentz, I. (2013). Hashimoto's Thyroiditis: Lifestyle Interventions for Finding and Treating the Root Cause. Des Plaines, IL: Wentz LLC.

Mind-Body Medicine

Gordon, J. S. (2008). Unstuck: Your Guide to the Seven-Stage Journey Out of Depression. New York, NY: Penguin Group.

Hay, L., Khadro, A., & Dane, H. (2015). Loving Yourself to Great Health: Thoughts & Food – The Ultimate Diet. Vista, CA: Hay House Inc.

Hyman, M. (2010). The UltraMind Solution: The Simple Way to Defeat Depression, Overcome Anxiety, and Sharpen Your Mind. New York, NY: Scribner.

Johnson, L. D. (2009). The Healing Power of Sleep!: A guide to healthy and refreshing sleep skills. Salt Lake City, UT: Head Acre Press.

McGonigal, K. (2012) The Willpower Instinct: How Self-Control Works, Why It Matters, and What You Can Do to Get More of It. New York, NY: Penguin Group.

McGonigal, K. (2015). The Upside of Stress: Why Stress is Good for You and How to Get Good At It. New York, NY: Penguin Group.

Minich, D. M. (2011). The Complete Handbook of Quantum Healing. San Francisco, CA: Conari Press.

Moss, D. P., McGrady, A. V., Davies, T. C., &
Wickramasekera, I. (2002). Handbook of Mind-Body
Medicine for Primary Care. Thousand Oaks, CA:
SAGE Publications, Inc.

Rankin, L. (2013). Mind Over Medicine: Scientific Proof
That You Can Heal Yourself. New York, NY: Hay
House, Inc.

Remen, R. N. (2006). Kitchen Table Wisdom. New York,
NY: Riverhead Books.

Sapolsky, R. (2004). Why Zebras Don't Get Ulcers. New
York, NY: Holt Paperbacks.

Nutrition

Ballantyle, S. (2014). The Paleo Approach: Reverse
Autoimmune Disease and Heal Your Body. Las
Vegas, NV: Victory Belt Publishing.

Bland, J. S. (2004). Clinical Nutrition: A Functional
Approach. Institute for Functional Medicine.

Davis, W. (2014). Wheat Belly: Lose the Wheat, Lose the
Weight, and Find Your Path Back to Health.
Emmaus, PA: Rodale Books.

Hooper, J. & Swift, K. M. (2014). The Swift Diet: 4 Weeks
to Mend the Belly, Lose the Weight, and Get Rid of
the Bloat. New York, NY: Hudson Street Press.

Junger, A. (2014). Clean Gut: The Breakthrough Plan for
Eliminating the Root Cause of Disease and
Revolutionizing Your Health. New York, NY:
HarperOne.

Linski, E. (2011). Digestive Wellness (4th ed.). New York,
NY: McGraw-Hill.

Ludwig, D. (2016). Always Hungry? Conquer Cravings,
Retrain Your Fat Cells, and Lose Weight
Permanently. London, UK: Orion Publishing Group.

Malterre, T. & Segersten, A. (2015). The Elimination Diet:
Discover the Foods That Are Making You Sick and
Tired—and Feel Better Fast. New York, NY: Grand
Central Life & Style.

Moss, M. (2014). Salt Sugar Fat: How the Food Giants Hooked Us. New York, NY: Random House Trade Paperbacks.

Mullin, G. (2015). The Gut Balance Revolution. New York, NY: Rodale Books.

Pitchford, P. (1996). Healing with Whole Foods: Oriental Traditions and Modern Nutrition. Berkeley, CA: North Atlantic Books.

Positive Psychology

Ben-Shahar, T. (2009). The Pursuit of Perfect: How to Stop Chasing Perfection and Start Living a Richer, Happier Life. New York, NY: McGraw-Hill Education.

Ben-Shahar, T. (2007). Happier: Learn the Secrets to Daily Joy and Lasting Fulfillment. New York, NY: McGraw-Hill Education.

Ben-Shahar, T. (2014). Choose the Life You Want: The Mindful Way to Happiness. New York, NY: The Experiment.

Biswas-Diener, R. & Kashdan, T. (2014). The Upside of Your Dark Side: Why Being Your Whole Self—Not Just Your "Good" Self—Drives Success and Fulfillment. New York, NY: Hudson Street Press.

Brown, B. (2010). The Gifts of Imperfection: Let Go of Who You Think You're Supposed to Be and Embrace Who You Are. Center City, MN: Hazelden Publishing.

Coelho, P. (2014). The Alchemist. San Francisco, CA: HarperOne.

Doman, F. (2016). Authentic Strengths. Las Vegas, NV: Next Century Publishing.

Duckworth, A. (2016). Grit: The Power of Passion and Perseverance. New York, NY: Scribner.

Emmons, H. & Kranz, R. (2006). The Chemistry of Joy: A Three-Step Program for Overcoming Depression Through Western Science and Eastern Wisdom. New York, NY: Touchstone.

Emmons, R. (2013). Gratitude Works! San Francisco, CA: Jossey-Bass.

Frankl, V. E. (2006). Man's Search for Meaning (Kindle Edition). Boston, MA: Beacon Press.

Fredrickson, B. (2013). Love 2.0: Creating Happiness and Health in Moments of Connection. New York, NY: Hudson Street Press.

Frisch, M. (2005). Quality of Life Therapy: Applying a Life Satisfaction Approach to Positive Psychology and Cognitive Therapy. Hoboken, NJ: Wiley and Sons.

Harvard Medical School. (2013). Positive Psychology: Harnessing the Power of Happiness, Mindfulness, and Inner Strength (Harvard Medical School Special Health Reports). Boston, MA: Harvard Health Publications.

Jacobs, B. & Jacobs, J. (2015). Life is Good: The Book – How to Live with Purpose & Enjoy the Ride. Washington, DC: National Geographic Society.

Johnson, L. (2007). Enjoy Life! Healing with Happiness. Head Acre Press.

Mehl-Madrona, L. (2010). Healing the Mind through the Power of Story: The Promise of Narrative Psychiatry. Rochester, VT: Bear and Company.

Miller, C. & Frisch, M. (2011). Creating Your Best Life. New York, NY: Sterling.

Niemiec, R. M. (2013). Mindfulness and Character Strengths. Boston, MA: Hogrefe Publishing.

Niemiec, R. M. & Wedding, D. (2014). Positive Psychology at the Movies. Boston, MA: Hogrefe Publishing.

Patterson, K., Grenny, J., Maxfield, D., McMillan, R., & Switzler, A. (2008). Influencer: The Power to Change Anything. New York, NY: McGraw-Hill Education.

Peterson, C. and Seligman, M (2004). Character Strengths and Virtues: A Handbook and Classification. Washington, DC: American Psychological Association/Oxford University Press.

Polly, S. & Britton, K. (2015). Character Strengths Matter: How to Live a Full Life. Minneapolis, MN: Graywolf Press.

Rafati, K. (2015). I Forgot to Die. Austin, TX: Lioncrest Publishing.

Rogers, C. R. (1995). On Becoming a Person: A Therapist's View of Psychotherapy. Boston: Houghton Mifflin.

Rollnick, S., Mason, P., & Butler, C. C. (1999). Health Behavior Change: A Guide for Practitioners (8th ed.). London, England: Churchill Livingstone.

Seligman, M. E. P. (2012). Flourish: A Visionary New Understanding of Happiness and Well- being. New York, NY: Free Press.

Seligman, M. E. P. (2014). Authentic Happiness. New York, NY: Atria Paperback.

Siegel, R. (2013). Positive Psychology: Harnessing the Power of Happiness, Mindfulness and Inner Strength (Harvard Medical School Special Health Reports). Boston, MA. Harvard Health Publications.

Sincero, J. (2013). You Are a Badass: How to Stop Doubting Your Greatness and Start Living an Awesome Life. Philadelphia, PA: Running Press.

Smith, E. E. (2017). The Power of Meaning: Crafting a Life That Matters. Danvers, MA: Crown Publishing.

Tarragona, M. (2013). Positive Identities: Narrative Practices and Positive Psychology. The Positive Psychology Workbook Series. Positive Acorn.

Virgin, J. J. (2017). Miracle Mindset: Show Up. Step Up. You are Stronger Than You Think. New York, NY: Simon and Schuster Digital Sales Inc.

Psychology of Eating

Chopra, D. (2014). What Are You Hungry For?: The Chopra Solution to Permanent Weight Loss. New York, NY: Harmony Books.

Kessler, D. (2010). The End of Overeating: Taking Control of the Insatiable American Appetite. Emmaus, PA: Rodale Books.

Miller, C. A. (2013). My Name is Caroline. Putnam Valley, NY: Cogent Publishing NY.

Miller, C. A. (2013). Positively Caroline: How I Beat Bulimia for Good and Found Real Happiness. Putnam Valley, NY: Cogent Publishing NY.

Rappoport, L. (2003). How We Eat: Appetite, Culture, and Psychology of Food. Toronto, Ontario: ECW Press.

Scott, T. (2011). The Anti-Anxiety Food Solution: How the Foods You Eat Can Help You Calm Your Anxious Mind, Improve Your Mood & End Cravings. Oakland, CA: New Harbinger Publications.

Taitz, J. L. (2012). End Emotional Eating: Using Dialectical Behavioral Therapy Skills to Cope With Difficult Emotions and Develop a Healthy Relationship to Food. Oakland, CA: New Harbinger Publications.

Wansink, B. (2006). Mindless Eating: Why We Eat More Than We Think. New York, NY: Bantam.

24337116R00099

Printed in Great Britain
by Amazon